QUESTIONS & ANSWERS ON

AIDS

LYN ROBERT FRUMKIN, M.D., Ph.D
Department of Neurology
University of California at Los Angeles

JOHN MARTIN LEONARD, M.D.
National Institute of Allergy and Infectious Diseases
National Institute of Health
Bethesda, Maryland

QUESTIONS & ANSWERS ON AIDS provides
factual information clearly and concisely written
in question-and-answer format.
Prepared by medical doctors for
health care professionals, patients, and families,
the responses are well considered,
well researched, and extremely current.

QUESTIONS & ANSWERS ON AIDS

AIDS

LYN FRUMKIN, M.D.
& JOHN LEONARD, M.D.

WITH A PREFACE BY
PAUL VOLBERDING, M.D., Ph.D.
& MICHAEL S. McGRATH, M.D., Ph.D.

AND A FOREWORD BY
ELISABETH KUBLER-ROSS, M.D.

 AVON
PUBLISHERS OF BARD, CAMELOT, DISCUS AND FLARE BOOKS

To Nadja, my wife, who helped inspire the project,
and to my parents, Joseph and Carol

—J.M.L.

To the memory of Herbert S. Ripley, MD,
physician, teacher, and friend

—L.R.F.

AVON BOOKS
A division of
The Hearst Corporation
105 Madison Avenue
New York, New York 10016

Copyright © 1987 by Lyn Robert Frumkin and John Martin Leonard
New foreword copyright © 1987 by Elisabeth Kubler-Ross
Published by arrangement with the authors
Library of Congress Catalog Card Number: 87-11288
ISBN: 0-380-75467-3

First Avon Printing: November 1987

AVON TRADEMARK REG. U.S. PAT. OFF. AND IN OTHER COUNTRIES, MARCA REGISTRADA, HECHO EN U.S.A.

Printed in the U.S.A.

K-R   10   9   8   7   6   5   4   3   2   1

Acknowledgments

We wish to thank our following friends and colleagues for their helpful comments and critical review: William Audeh, MD, Ann Collier, MD, Read Handyside, Tara Hawkins, Katherine Knowles, William Hanson, MD, R. James Kellogg, Minna Levitt, William Lutge, MD, Kenneth Melmon, MD, John Sotos, MD, CarolAnn Stockton and Shiurah Vollmer, MD. Marla Frumkin, Peter Stelzer, and Nadja Leonard deserve special appreciation for their comments, encouragement, and support. At all times they have shared our desire to provide a book that could help the reader to better understand the acquired immunodeficiency syndrome.

The people showed a great concern at this, and began to be alarmed all over town, and the more, because in the last week of December 1664 another man died in the same house and of the same distemper. And then we were easy again for about six weeks, when none having died with any marks of infection, it was said the distemper was gone; but after that, I think it was about the 12th of February, another died in another house, but in the same parish and in the same manner.

Daniel Defoe, London, 1722
A Journal of the Plague Year

AIDS is a life-threatening disease and a major public health issue. Its impact on our society is and will continue to be devastating. By the end of 1991, an estimated 270,000 cases of AIDS will have occurred with 179,000 deaths within the decade since the disease was first recognized . . . [and] the number of people estimated to be [presently] infected with the AIDS virus in the United States is about 1.5 million.

C. Everett Koop, MD, 1986
Surgeon General's Report on
Acquired Immune Deficiency Syndrome

Contents

A Note from the Authors   xiv

Foreword by Elisabeth Kubler-Ross, MD   xv

Preface by Michael S. McGrath, MD, PhD,
and Paul A. Volberding, MD, PhD   xvii

Introduction   xix

CHAPTER ONE
What Is AIDS?
Definitions and the Origin of the Syndrome   1

Initial Reported Cases · Opportunistic
Infection · Immune System and Lymphocytes   1

Definitions of Terms: Acquired and Transmissible,
Immunity, Syndrome   2

Original Definition of AIDS   4

Viruses · Diseases Caused by
Viruses · Mechanisms of Action of
Viruses · Retroviruses · T and B
Lymphocytes · Action of AIDS Virus   4

Replacement of Lymphocytes as
Therapy · Antiviral Drugs · Vaccines   7

Simian Immunodeficiency Syndrome · Origin of
New Viruses · Speculation on Origin of AIDS   10

CHAPTER TWO
How AIDS Manifests Itself:
The Five Principal AIDS-Related Conditions   13

*AIDS, AIDS-Related Complex (ARC), Generalized
Lymphadenopathy Syndrome (GLS), Antibody
Positivity, and Acute Infection*   13

*AIDS: Symptoms · Sites and Types of
Infections · Most Common Infection · Kaposi's
Sarcoma · Prognosis and Quality of Life · Affinity
of AIDS Virus for Nervous System
Cells · Significance of Ability of AIDS Virus to
Infect Brain Tissue · Factors Affecting
Mortality · Expansion of Definition of AIDS*   14

*AIDS-Related Complex (ARC):
Definition · Prognosis · Relation to AIDS*   23

*Generalized Lymphadenopathy Syndrome
(GLS): Definition · Prognosis · Relation to AIDS*   25

Antibody Positivity: Definition · Prognosis   26

Acute Infection: Definition · Prognosis   27

*Interrelationship of All AIDS-Related
Conditions · Interval of Time between Infection
and Symptoms of AIDS · Current CDC
Classification of AIDS-Related Conditions*   27

CHAPTER THREE
Who Gets AIDS? Groups at Risk   30

*Number of Children and Adults with
AIDS · Percentages of Persons with AIDS Who
Are Homosexual Men, Intravenous Drug Abusers,
Blood Transfusion Recipients, Hemophiliacs,
Heterosexual Partners of Persons with AIDS or at
High Risk, and Pesons Not in Known Risk Groups*   30

CHAPTER FOUR
**How AIDS Is Acquired:
Modes of Transmissibility**   32

*Homosexuals · Blood and Semen
Transmission · Oral and Rectal Sex · Lesbians*   34

Contents

Heterosexuals and AIDS   34

Prisoners   35

*Heterosexual Female-to-Male
Transmission · Female Prostitutes · Percentage of
Heterosexual-to-Total Cases of
AIDS · Asymptomatic Carriers of AIDS Virus*   36

Intravenous Drug Abusers   38

*Children and Infants with AIDS · Risk to a Child
from Breast Feeding by an Infected
Mother · Recommendations for Routine
Vaccinations in an Infected Child*   39

*Casual Contact, Saliva, and Transmission of
AIDS · AIDS in Persons Not in Known Risk
Groups*   43

Hemophiliacs   45

*Risk of Acquiring AIDS by Hepatitis B
Vaccine · Risk of Acquiring AIDS by
Immunoglobulin Injections · Risk of Acquiring
AIDS by Blood Protein Injections · Summary of
Ways AIDS Can Be Transmitted through Blood-
Borne Routes*   48

*Those Who Should Refrain from Blood
Donation · Risk of Acquiring AIDS through Blood
Donation and Insect Bites · Persons in Nonrisk
Groups Acquiring AIDS*   50

Haitians   52

CHAPTER FIVE
**Exposure to the AIDS Virus:
The Meaning of Antibody Positivity**   54

*Meaning of Blood Donation Screening to Detect
Exposure to AIDS Virus · Risk of Acquiring AIDS
through Donation of Blood · Incidence of Infected
Blood in Blood Bank Testing · Notification of*

*Those Donating Blood Who Test Antibody
Positive · Further Evaluation of Individuals
Whose Blood Tests Antibody Positive · Locations
Besides Blood Donation Centers to Have Antibody
Status Determined*   54

*Use of Screening Test to Detect AIDS Virus
Exposure · Types, Accuracy, Limitations, and
Nature of Tests · Summary of Meaning of Testing
Antibody Positive*   56

*Limitations to a Mass Screening
Program · Antibody Negativity and Antibody
Negativity in Persons with AIDS · Time Period
between Infection and Demonstration of Antibody
Positivity · General Value of Testing · Infectivity
of Antibody Positive Persons · Antibody
Negativity and Infectivity · Ability of Antibody
Test to Predict Occurrence of Disease*   58

*Recommendations for Antibody Positive Persons
to Decrease Risk of Infecting
Others · Recommendations to Infected Women for
Family Planning · Pregnancy as a Risk Factor
for Acquiring AIDS in the Infected
Woman · Antibody Screening as a Part of the
Premarital Blood Screen · Antibody Positivity as
an Indicator of Decreased Immune Functioning*   65

*Life Insurance and Antibody Positivity · Table of
Prevalence of Antibody Positivity in Different
Groups · Military Use of Antibody Positivity
Screening · Groups That Should Have Antibody
Testing*   68

*Recommendations to Decrease Risk of Acquiring
AIDS · Changes in Sexual Behavior of
Homosexuals and Heterosexuals · Use of
Condoms and Other Devices as
Protection · Recommendations Regarding Sex
between Two Infected Persons*   70

Contents

CHAPTER SIX
Protecting the Individual and Health Care Worker

75

Risk to Health Care Workers of Acquiring AIDS or Infection in the Workplace · Risk of Acquiring AIDS or Infection to Household Members Caring for Persons with AIDS · Prevention of AIDS and Infection in Health Care Workers and Others Caring for AIDS Patients · Accidental Stick by Needle Used in the Care of an AIDS Patient   75

Infectivity of and Exposure to Tears · Legality of Requiring Patient to Undergo Antibody Testing · Risk of Acquiring AIDS from Salivary Exchange through CPR Courses and Mouth-to-Mouth Resuscitation · Saliva and Sharing of Food Utensils · Role of Food-Service Workers in Transmission of AIDS   77

Artificial Insemination and Risk of Acquiring AIDS   80

Means of Disinfecting Contaminated External Surfaces, Linens, and Medical Instruments   80

Effect of Factors Known to Decrease Immunity on Risk of Acquiring AIDS · Pregnancy and Risks Involved through the Care of Persons with AIDS · Organ Transplant Recipients · Other Practices Capable of Transmitting the AIDS Virus   81

Table Summarizing the Type of Body Secretion, Presence or Absence of Virus, and Possible Modes of Transmissibility   83

Recommendations Regarding AIDS and Infectivity in Children and Attendance at School · Response of Communities to Such Recommendations   84

Quarantining · Legality of Terminating Employment of a Person with AIDS · Legality of AIDS as a Protected Handicap · Legality of

*Employers Requiring Antibody Testing of Job
Applicants and Employees · Publications on
Legal Aspects of AIDS*   87

CHAPTER SEVEN
The Epidemiology of AIDS   93

*AIDS Epidemic and Pandemic · Areas of the
World Affected by AIDS · Prevalence of AIDS in
Non-U.S. Countries · Significance of African
Epidemiological Patterns to the U.S. · CDC
Redefinition of AIDS for Underdeveloped
Countries without Antibody Testing
Facilities · Measures Non-U.S. Countries Are
Taking to Limit Spread of AIDS · Geographic
Distribution of U.S. Cases*   93

*Risk of Acquiring AIDS for a Person without
Known Risk Factors · Mortality Figure for
AIDS · Future Growth Patterns · Economic Costs
of AIDS · Alternate Sites of Care for Persons with
AIDS*   100

CHAPTER EIGHT
Research and Funding for AIDS   105

*Amount of Money Appropriated for AIDS
Research · Where the Funds Go · Comparison of
Amount Appropriated for AIDS with That for
Other Research Purposes*   105

*Experimental Drugs and Modes of Action · FDA
Approval · Other Developments Important to
AIDS Research · Speed and Procedures for FDA
Approval of Experimental Drugs*   106

*Location of Centers for AIDS Research · AIDS
Funding by Private Foundations · Where to Send
Donations for AIDS Research and Patient
Care · Federal Assistance Programs for Persons
with AIDS*   110

CHAPTER NINE
Resource Centers for AIDS Information and Support 113

List of National and Local Centers 113

Where Physicians Report Cases of AIDS · Free Pamphlets Providing Basic Information on AIDS · Sources of Scientific Literature on AIDS 127

CHAPTER TEN
Epilogue 130

Ethical and Social Dilemmas of the AIDS Crisis · Approach of Ethicists to These Dilemmas · Attitudes of Americans to Social Issues Surrounding AIDS 130

Preferences of Persons with AIDS for Life-Sustaining Treatments · The Physician's Responsibility to an AIDS Patient 132

What Medicine Has Learned from the Study of AIDS 134

Perspectives 136

Glossary 138

References 152

Index 199

A Note from the Authors

The idea to write this book originated from the countless questions posed to us by friends, patients, families of patients, and health professionals during our training as housestaff physicians at Stanford. Our perception at that time was that there was a lack of easy-to-read, accessible literature that would enable health care workers to acquire general but comprehensive information about AIDS. We undertook this project at a time when almost daily reports from television and the popular press reflected a hunger for additional information of social, ethical, legal, and medical importance on AIDS. It is our experience that the need and demand for information on AIDS has increased with each passing month.

We have chosen a question-and-answer approach as the best way to balance what we hoped would be a readable format with one sophisticated enough to incorporate both necessary detail and accuracy. Our goal is to educate the health care worker by answering questions we imagine might arise concerning AIDS. We appreciate, however, that much remains to be learned before the final word on AIDS is in.

L.R.F.
J.M.L.

June 1, 1987

Foreword

AIDS first appeared in the United States several years ago and, although initially the significance was not fully appreciated, it soon became evident that this disease was more than just a new medical syndrome. As reports of cases started to accumulate, an alarm began to ring in many places that AIDS was to become one of the greatest national, if not world, health issues of the present time.

Drs. Frumkin and Leonard's *Questions & Answers on AIDS* is a welcome addition to the ever-increasing literature on AIDS which has sprung up in the past few years. It is a meticulous collection of the myriad of issues facing this epidemic, addressed not only to caregivers, but also to the healthy infected person, the AIDS patient, and his or her family. In addition to the person with AIDS, those caring for the affected person are also in need of an accurate understanding of the illness and emotional support to best prepare for a lengthy and often lonely vigil at the bedside of a dying adult or child.

Anyone afraid of AIDS should read this book, which is written in an objective and understandable fashion. All people, however, whether caregivers or not, need to know that they cannot contract AIDS by casual contact and this book will help them appreciate that. It will also minimize the pathological fear that millions have expressed toward those either with AIDS or infected with the AIDS virus. If individuals can also detach themselves from their own panic, reading this book may enlighten many who will then be ready to "pitch in" and help their fellow man.

With the doubling of AIDS cases every ten months, it is mandatory that we prepare ourselves now and not tomorrow. This can be done, in part, by recruiting a generation of volunteers and health care workers willing to staff hospices for adults and children with this deadly disease. We can also minimize costly hospital stays, which persons with AIDS can least afford, by working to create alternatives for housing those who are not in need of an acute hospital setting. With many AIDS patients currently being cared for in hospital rooms at a cost of $600–1000 per day, such alternatives will slow the financial burden this disease has placed on our total health care system.

AIDS is more than just a disease, it is a phenomenon that brings into the open our "dis-ease": our own fears, prejudices, and needs to blame, judge, and criticize others. Although many choose to see AIDS as a disease affecting primarily homosexual men, it is a terminal illness affecting thousands from all walks of life. AIDS is an ultimate challenge to a society rarely faced with a disease that has raised as great a degree of psychological, social, legal, and ethical dilemmas. The fact that AIDS mainly affects young adults and children provokes even more fear and anguish, in proportions far greater than the social turmoil that surrounded the dreaded leprosy of Father Damien's time.

Let your friends and neighbors read this book, and discuss with each other its implications. Make it an issue to share it with your children, so they too can express their feelings and consider accepting a hemophiliac child with AIDS to their classroom and playground. This is your chance to base your understanding and decisions on knowledge and not on fear. I thank Drs. Frumkin and Leonard for sharing this meaningful information with the many who will read it.

Elisabeth Kubler-Ross, MD
Headwaters, Virginia

Preface

In only a short period of time AIDS has become a household word across the United States. Rapid advances in the fields of immunology and virology have identified the etiologic agent of AIDS as a virus. Although scientists across the world have made many important discoveries about the AIDS virus and its role in causing AIDS, the development of truly effective therapies and vaccines is likely to take many years. In the absence of readily available, highly effective treatment for AIDS, the only way that we can hope to control the spread of AIDS is through extensive educational efforts.

As the AIDS epidemic has increased in numbers and as additional groups have been affected, there has been a commensurate increase in questions from medical providers and the general public about the nature of this epidemic. This book, *Questions & Answers on AIDS*, provides factual information in response to the many questions being asked. The book is clearly and concisely written and is presented in a question-and-answer format. In response to the questions ranging from the basic biology of the human immunodeficiency virus to the epidemiology of the epidemic to the care and prevention of the disease, the authors provide well considered responses. These responses are extremely current and well researched, yet presented in a very readable style and format. In addition, the authors include a very useful glossary of terms which should be of particular value to the reader not well versed in AIDS, and a list of resources for further information which should be used by all levels of readers.

Preface

This book, *Questions & Answers on AIDS,* fills a very large void in our widening array of educational materials concerning this epidemic. The authors have done an extremely commendable job and this book will be a valuable resource to many.

Paul A. Volberding, MD, PhD
Chief, AIDS Activities Division
UCSF-San Francisco General Hospital

Michael S. McGrath, MD, PhD
Director
AIDS Immunobiology Research Laboratory
UCSF-San Francisco General Hospital

Introduction

In 1981, a cluster of homosexual men were identified who had unexplainable, typically fatal infections. The severity of infections in these men reflected a failure of their immune system to fight off invading microorganisms that generally pose no threat to the average person. In addition, the inability to fight off infection in these men was underscored by the fact that these individuals had not received drugs nor had diseases known to affect normal immunity. What was initially perceived as a phenomenon limited only to homosexual men quickly expanded to include intravenous drug abusers who used nonsterile needles and some recipients of blood transfusions. The spread of the illness to these latter two groups suggested that the cause of the disease was an agent transmitted through both blood and semen. It was at this time that the term *Acquired Immunodeficiency Syndrome*, or AIDS, was coined. It described an acquired disease of the immune system that reflected a deficiency in immunity and predisposed affected persons to frequent and overwhelming infections. Less than three years later, researchers isolated a virus as the causative agent. By that time, over 12,000 Americans had contracted the disease. Most of those affected died within a year of diagnosis, and it was estimated that the number of cases would double each eight to ten months.

We now know what causes AIDS, how it is transmitted, and who is at risk. The AIDS virus predisposes its host to infection with many organisms by killing lymphocytes, cells in the bloodstream crucial to the body's ability to fight off invading bacteria, fungi, protozoa, and viruses. Although found in a variety of body fluids, the virus is principally transmitted through sexual contact and the sharing of intravenous needles. We also now recognize that AIDS is only one condition in a spectrum of transmissible immunodeficiency diseases involving the AIDS virus. There are, for example, up to 1.5 million people who have been infected with the virus but who have no symptoms, as well as those who have symptoms less devastating than seen in fully developed cases of AIDS. Regardless of the presence or absence of symptoms, each of these persons is regarded as carrying the virus and as being capable of infecting others who, in turn, may develop any of the known AIDS syndromes.

The recognition that infected individuals, whether heterosexual or homosexual, male or female, can carry the virus and transmit it to others without developing symptoms or knowing that they are carriers has raised public debate over the proper use of screening tests to detect the presence of the AIDS virus. These tests, which have limitations, have been proposed for use in screening military recruits, life insurance applicants, and persons from high-risk groups such as those who share intravenous needles or who have many sexual partners. How should the results of these tests be interpreted? What is the risk of acquiring AIDS in those who have prior exposure to and infection with the virus? What is the relation between the isolation of the AIDS virus in blood, semen, saliva, tears, and breast milk of infected individuals and its transmissibility to others? How can infected persons reduce their risk of infecting others—and what recommendations exist to decrease the risk to a noninfected person of acquiring AIDS or being exposed to the AIDS virus? If the AIDS virus is found in saliva, why has casual contact not been considered a method of AIDS transmissibility? What is suggested regarding the consideration of pregnancy if a person has no symptoms but is infected with the AIDS virus? How can a heterosexual person without symptoms of disease transmit AIDS to another heterosexual individual? These are questions that have been posed to us and are answerable within the framework of what is currently known about AIDS.

CHAPTER ONE

What Is AIDS?
Definitions and the
Origin of the Syndrome

1. How was AIDS first discovered in the United States?

In mid-1981, unusual opportunistic infections began to occur in homosexual men and users of intravenous drugs. The infections proved to be uniformly fatal and unprecedented in severity in these previously healthy individuals. This apparently new condition was named the Acquired Immunodeficiency Syndrome, or AIDS. Although it first attracted limited attention, an *ABC News* and *Washington Post* poll demonstrated that by 1985 Americans perceived AIDS as only slightly lower than cancer as the nation's biggest health problem. This rapid increase in awareness of AIDS has fueled a sense of urgency as the medical and lay communities have sought how best to deal with the rising incidence of this dreaded and often poorly understood disease.

2. What are opportunistic infections?

Infection occurs when a microorganism such as a virus, bacterium, fungus, or protozoan invades another organism and disease is produced. There are many microorganisms that we are exposed to daily but produce no disease in healthy individuals. When our immunity or natural ability to resist disease is lessened, such as occurs in some patients receiving chemotherapy or those born with rare defects in immunity, these normally benign microorganisms become "opportunistic" and can then cause severe infection and fatal disease.

3. What normally makes humans immune to disease?

Our immune system is made up of cells and specific proteins in our blood that recognize and initiate reactions to destroy invading organisms. Two critical elements of our immune system are the cellular component, with the lymphocytes playing an especially important role, and the protein component, which includes the antibodies.

4. So, what is AIDS?

AIDS is an acronym for Acquired Immunodeficiency Syndrome. Immunodeficiency refers to the inability of the immune system to function properly, thus making the individual susceptible to a variety of infections not typically found in the immunologically normal person.

5. And, what is meant by the terms "acquired" and "syndrome"?

In mid-1981, the Centers for Disease Control (CDC) in Atlanta, Georgia, a federal agency concerned with monitoring disease frequency, began receiving reports from physicians of unusual opportunistic infections in homosexual men and intravenous drug users. Because a wide range of opportunistic infections can occur when immunity is severely decreased, there was no characteristic set of physical signs or symptoms that was, by itself, diagnostic of AIDS. There was instead a group of signs and symptoms that reflected immunodeficiency in affected persons who otherwise had no known reasons to have disorders of immunity. That group of signs and symptoms was designated the Acquired Immunodeficiency Syndrome, or AIDS.

A constellation of findings comprises a syndrome even though the findings may not be identical in any two people. For example, while a homosexual patient may develop an unexplained deficiency in immunity that is manifested as pneumonia, that same syndrome may become manifest in an intravenous drug abuser as a brain infection. Both individuals —with different opportunistic infections and not taking drugs or sick with diseases that can drastically compromise one's immune system—can be said to have the same "immunodeficiency syndrome."

6. But what about the term "acquired"?

As reports of this immunodeficiency syndrome among homosexual individuals and intravenous drug users accumulated, it became apparent that the pattern of appearance of this disease was suggestive of a transmissible disease. The disease seemed to be spread through contact with semen or blood.

During the initial period of recognition of this syndrome, attempts were made to better define the nature of the disease by comparing homosexual men with AIDS to homosexual men without AIDS. The most important difference between these two groups was that the ill patients had a significantly greater number of sexual partners in the preceding year compared with the healthy group. Thus, the notion of this syndrome as a sexually transmissible "acquired" illness began to develop. The hypothesis of a transmissible acquired disease received further support with the occurrence of the syndrome in individuals who had received transfusions with blood products. This showed that the disease could also be acquired from some agent in blood.

7. So, "acquired" really means "transmissible"?

In this case, yes. We are familiar with a wide range of acquired diseases caused by contact with transmitted viruses, bacteria, and other microorganisms. These include the virally caused "common cold" and hepatitis B, fungus-induced "athlete's foot," and a countless number of illnesses related to bacterial infections such as impetigo, various pneumonias, bronchitis, and conjunctivitis. Acquired, therefore, implies the acquisition of a disease that a person would not have contracted if contact with the responsible agent had not occurred. Thus, acquired serves to distinguish a process that develops as a result of some influence outside the body from a genetic process with which a person may be born.

8. Can the original definition of AIDS be paraphrased?

AIDS or Acquired Immunodeficiency Syndrome is a fatal illness that (1) is acquired; (2) occurs in those individuals whose immune systems were previously normal but have become severely deficient; (3) is characterized by a group of symptoms and signs that may differ from person to person, but result from opportunistic infections with microorganisms that produce no disease in normal people. In addition, because of an unusually high incidence in homosexual men of the previously rare cancer, Kaposi's sarcoma, the presence of this malignancy was also considered evidence of AIDS, even in the absence of an opportunistic infection.

According to criteria outlined by the CDC, individuals must also be younger than 60 years old, not have received immunosuppressive drugs, and have no other apparent immunosuppressive disease. The presence of opportunistic infections in the elderly population, while rare, resulted in the above criterion to distinguish AIDS from a possible age-related immunodeficiency.

9. If the agent causing AIDS is transmissible, what is it?

A virus.

10. What is a virus?

Viruses are microorganisms that are usually composed of a protein coat that encases a core of the nucleic acids RNA or DNA. RNA and DNA are the chemical constituents of genes in all organisms. Viruses typically range in size from 10 to 250 nanometers (1 nanometer is 1 billionth of a meter).

These small agents are capable of infecting almost all members of the plant and animal kingdoms, including bacteria. Viruses are dependent on their hosts for reproduction because they lack an independent metabolism and are unable to grow on their own. As such, viruses have alternately been characterized as both living objects and inert chemicals. Both characterizations are semantically correct depending upon different biological perspectives.

11. Can viruses be seen?

Under the optical microscopes with which most are familiar, viruses are too small to be seen. However, highly specialized electron microscopes have been developed that can take pictures of viruses and demonstrate detail as much as 10,000 times finer than obtained with optical microscopes. In addition, many viruses can be grown, crystallized, and have their structure deduced by biochemical techniques.

12. What types of diseases do viruses cause in humans?

The viruses that cause diseases come from many subtypes or families. They are responsible for as diverse a group of illnesses as the common cold, herpes, chicken pox, mononucleosis, mumps, warts, and perhaps some cancers.

13. What type of virus is the AIDS virus?

There are many different types of viruses that, like animals, bacteria, and plants, may be grouped together on the basis of increasing similarities. In late 1983 and early 1984, very similar viruses were independently isolated from patients with AIDS at the Pasteur Institute in Paris and at the National Institutes of Health (NIH) in Washington, DC. These two viruses were retroviruses, belonging to the family of viruses that contain principally RNA as their core nucleic acid. Retroviruses are sensitive to destruction by ether, have a diameter of around 100 nanometers, have a characteristic life cycle, and have been identified as the causative agents for a variety of tumors and syndromes of immunosuppression in animals.

Many viruses display "tropism," or a preference for a specific tissue as their site of infection. Because the preferred site of infection by the AIDS virus is the T-lymphocyte cell of the immune system, the American research group called their virus *HTLV-III* (Human T-Cell Lymphotropic Virus-III). The French team called their virus *LAV,* or Lymphadenopathy-Associated Virus, referring to the nonspecific symptoms of enlarged lymph nodes (lymphadenopathy) initially noted in many persons with AIDS.

Because the AIDS virus has appeared in the literature under the names HTLV-III/LAV, HTLV-III, LAV, and ARV (AIDS-Associated Retrovirus), an international committee of virologists voted in early 1986 to recommend that scientists use the term HIV (Human Immunodeficiency Virus) when referring to the causative agent of AIDS. HIV is becoming the most widely accepted name, although the terms HTLV-III/LAV, HTLV-III, LAV, and ARV are still used by some scientists and writers when referring to the virus that causes AIDS.

14. How is it known that this virus causes AIDS?

Isolating the virus from a person with AIDS is not in itself adequate to determine that the virus is the causative agent for AIDS. Conclusive proof would come from recreating the illness in a normal human by administering the virus to that individual. Although one cannot ethically inoculate individuals in an attempt to reproduce this illness, there are a variety of other means that allow scientists to draw strong conclusions regarding causality.

First, the virus is only rarely seen in nature and when found it is often associated with some manifestation of AIDS. Additionally, most persons with AIDS have had blood tests suggesting exposure to the virus at some time in the course of their illness. There are cases from the period prior to the use of screening tests for exposure to the virus in which the administration of blood later shown to contain HIV led to the development of AIDS in the recipient patients. This situation actually simulates administering the virus to a previously uninfected person and then having that person contract AIDS. Finally, in test tube settings, the virus has been shown to infect and destroy lymphocytes, thereby mimicking the process that occurs in the body.

15. What is a lymphocyte?

It is a type of blood cell. Lymphocytes comprise a class of white blood cells that has as one of its functions the resistance to infection. The lymphocytes are composed of two major groups: the B-lymphocytes and the T-lymphocytes. B-lymphocytes secrete proteins called antibodies that are important for neutralizing foreign substances in the blood, such as invading microorganisms. T-lymphocytes have many functions, one of which is the direct attack on many different microorganisms. Other specialized blood cells among the lymphocytes are capable of killing both tumor and infected cells. It is a subtype of the class of T-lymphocytes—the helper T-lymphocytes, otherwise called T_4 lymphocytes—that the AIDS virus specifically infects and kills. This infection renders the body unable to mount a normal response to infecting microorganisms.

16. How does the AIDS virus decrease a person's immunity to fight infection?

The AIDS virus has an affinity for lymphocytes, which are a crucial component of the immune system. After the T_4 lymphocyte population is substantially depleted by the AIDS virus, patients develop the clinical signs of AIDS. Persons with AIDS not only have a decrease in their blood-borne helper T-lymphocytes, but also have accompanying increases in a cell type that suppresses helper T-lymphocyte activity. These cells are called suppressor-cytotoxic T-lymphocytes. Thus, persons with AIDS have a marked alteration of the T-lymphocyte helper: suppressor ratio, an important indicator of immune competence in patients. In normal individuals, this ratio is greater than 1.7; in persons with AIDS, this ratio is usually less than 0.9, and often less than 0.5.

The mechanism by which the AIDS virus decreases immunity has also been suggested by test tube models of the infection. When T-lymphocytes are removed from infected persons and placed in specially prepared cultures outside the body, these cells rapidly die and release the AIDS virus. Cell death in culture usually occurs two to three weeks after infection. Recent experiments suggest that some surviving lymphocytes, not necessarily the T_4 type, continue to harbor the virus indefinitely and may serve as a reservoir for the virus.

17. Why not just replace the lymphocytes to cure AIDS?

We know that the virus infects and kills the helper T-lymphocytes. However, a host of other immunological abnormalities also exists, including excessive, nonspecific activation of the antibody-producing B-lymphocytes, altered levels of an antiviral protein called interferon, decreased ability of various types of lymphocytes to destroy a foreign agent, and weakened ability of lymphocytes in general to move toward an invading agent or microorganism. It would seem likely, therefore, that simply transfusing T-lymphocytes into an AIDS patient would still leave a number of immunological problems unresolved and lead to a continued decrease in immune system competence. Reconstitution of the immune system by infusing chemicals including the immune stimulants interferon and interleukin-2 has been attempted. This approach has proved ineffective in altering the course of the disease.

Because the bone marrow is the site of production of lymphocytes in healthy individuals, an even more aggressive approach to "reconstitute" the immune system has been attempted with bone marrow transplantation in an AIDS patient. The patient had a small increase in T-cells with a partial recovery of some of his previously missing immune functions. Unfortunately, these benefits were transient. The failure of aggressive treatment in the form of bone marrow transplantation illustrates the difficulty of lymphocyte replacement in patients who most likely continue to harbor the virus at other sites within their bodies. Without effective antiviral agents that can rid the host of the virus, the artificial infusion of new lymphocytes does not appear to be a viable therapeutic option.

18. Why can't the scientific community find a drug to kill the AIDS virus?

There are no antiviral drugs that can control a disease by killing an infecting virus. Consider how drugs to destroy or limit bacterial growth have been developed. Bacteria are infinitely more complex than viruses; the smallest bacterium is still larger than the biggest virus. Structurally, bacteria resemble animal cells in having the internal machinery necessary to grow, reproduce, and exist independently of other cells. Thus, bacteria are similar to animal cells in many ways. However, bacteria also differ from animal cells in several simple but crucial ways. In contrast to animal cells, for example, certain bacteria possess a rigid cell wall that contains a unique chemical structure. Penicillin is an example of an antibiotic or antibacterial drug that selectively inhibits or "poisons" bacterial cell wall synthesis. The susceptibility of a bacterium to penicillin, therefore, is in part determined by the bacterium's structure that is both unique and complex enough to differentiate it from animal cells and allow selective destruction. There are many different antibiotics because there are many ways in which different bacterial cells are unique in comparison to animal cells and therefore susceptible to selective poisoning that leaves host cells unharmed.

Unfortunately, few drugs selectively poison viruses. Because viruses lack the complicated internal machinery of bacterial cells necessary for independent existence and survival, they are not susceptible to antibiotics useful against other organisms. While it is true that most viruses can be destroyed by heat, cold, radiation, and chemicals such as ether and formaldehyde, these processes also destroy animal cells and offer no selective destruction of viruses.

19. Why, then, have viral diseases such as polio been drastically reduced and some such as smallpox eradicated?

Vaccines have been developed against these viruses. The immune system includes lymphocytes and antibodies that destroy microorganisms introduced into the body. These cells and proteins recognize a virus, bacterium, or other organism as foreign by the unique chemical structure (like a fingerprint) of the microorganism and are able to mount an immune response. This immune response consists of an increased number either of lymphocytes, antibodies, or both that can destroy the offending agent.

A vaccine can be a virus or component of a virus that has been chemically or otherwise altered in such a way as to lose its disease-producing properties while still retaining enough of its unique chemical structure to be able to evoke an immune response in the host. The immune response that results from the vaccine is able to protect the host from the live virus. Thus, vaccines have the advantage of acting like the natural infection with regard to their effect on immunity; they stimulate long-lasting resistance to the microorganism by causing the individual to accumulate specific antibodies and "memory cells" that can quickly mount an immune response when re-challenged by an exposure to the virus.

The development of a vaccine assumes that the part of the virus used to stimulate an immune response has been rendered unable to cause disease. Vaccines have been developed for a wide range of viral diseases, including polio, mumps, rubella, smallpox, and hepatitis B.

20. Why is such a vaccine not available against the AIDS virus?

There are many reasons why a vaccine is not yet available. First, the disease is newly described; scientists have known the causative agent and have been convinced of its role only since 1984. Vaccines are also difficult to construct and ade-quately test. For example, before a vaccine can safely be ad-ministered to a population, it must be demonstrated that the vaccine itself will not cause disease. The AIDS virus has a longer incubation period (time between infection and onset of symptoms) than other viral diseases which makes the assess-ment of vaccine effectiveness and safety difficult. In addition, the chemical composition of the AIDS virus coat is highly variable and appears to change rapidly. This variability sug-gests that a vaccine protecting against one strain of AIDS virus may not provide immunity against others.

21. Is AIDS a truly new disease?

There is no known precedent for AIDS in recorded human medicine. Unusual cancers caused by retroviruses have been identified in the last decade, but the scope, rapidity of spread, clinical presentation, and the newly described causative agent make AIDS unique.

22. Is there any disease similar to AIDS?

A syndrome called Simian Acquired Immunodeficiency Syn-drome (SAIDS), closely resembling human AIDS in its presentation, has been described in the macaque monkey. It is endemic in several primate centers in the United States. This syndrome has been shown to result from infection with a type D retrovirus, an agent that is similar in some respects to the AIDS virus. Perhaps most importantly for the study of AIDS, two lymphotropic human viruses, called HTLV-4 and LAV-2, have been isolated from persons in Western Africa. The exact relation of these two viruses to the AIDS virus and their ability to produce disease remains to be determined.

23. How do new viruses first appear in nature?

It is unlikely that new viruses appear without being derived first from some other related virus. There are clear examples throughout biology in which viruses are able to change their shape, size, infectivity, and other less dramatic functions, thereby providing means for the creation of new variations. Viruses do change continuously and, given sufficient time, later generations of viruses may be very different from their ancestors.

24. Which viruses change?

All viruses will change over time. The most classic example is the virus causing influenza, or "flu." The virus is able to change the chemical composition of its protein coat yearly. Even after developing influenza, a person remains susceptible to the virus when it reappears covered by a new coat no longer recognized by the antibodies from the last infection. When enough people are susceptible and the virus has radically changed, then an epidemic of influenza is possible from the new virus. The AIDS virus also presumably evolved from a related virus existing elsewhere in nature.

25. What are the current ideas about the origin of the AIDS virus?

Scientists can only speculate as to how the AIDS virus came about and where it first appeared. There are, however, some good clues. As mentioned, an AIDS-like virus causing Simian Acquired Immunodeficiency Syndrome in monkeys has been isolated. A different retrovirus related to HIV has been isolated recently from wild African Green monkeys. Careful review of illnesses occurring in Central Africa has found cases of unexplained opportunistic infections in patients as early as 1975 that today would meet the current CDC definiton of AIDS. It seems likely that the current epidemic may have first occurred somewhere in Central Africa in the mid-1970s.

While it is probably true that we will never know the circumstances surrounding the first case, some scientists have argued that the virus might have been originally present in monkeys in the distant past and later escaped that host. Researchers have found lymphotropic human viruses that seem to be intermediate between the Simian viruses and the virus causing AIDS in humans. This adds further support to the idea that the AIDS virus may have originated from intermediate human viruses not presently known to be associated with disease which were descendants of the virus found in monkeys.

CHAPTER TWO

How AIDS Manifests Itself: The Five Principal AIDS-Related Conditions

26. So, it is now understood that AIDS is a newly discovered, transmissible disease caused by a virus. What are the symptoms of AIDS?

Because AIDS is a disease in which immunodeficiency is the underlying problem, the symptoms of AIDS differ among individuals, reflecting the specific underlying opportunistic infection. Those with AIDS are susceptible to a wide range of opportunistic infections, be they viral, bacterial, fungal, or protozoan. In addition, persons with AIDS have an unusually high incidence of both Kaposi's sarcoma, a previously rare cancer, and neurological disease unrelated to opportunistic infections.

A wide variety of manifestations of AIDS virus infection have been recognized. A transient illness characterized by fever, enlarged lymph nodes, malaise, sore muscles, diarrhea, skin rash, and a sore throat has been described in a number of persons within days to weeks after AIDS virus exposure. Although these symptoms are characteristic of many different types of viral infections such as the common cold or flu, they represent an initial response to infection with the AIDS virus. Some, but not all, of the individuals who start with these nonspecific symptoms go on to have the severe infections and/or Kaposi's sarcoma that characterizes AIDS.

The early term *Gay Lymphadenopathy Syndrome* came into being to describe the earliest reports of additional persons who had lymphadenopathy, or enlarged lymph nodes, associated with complaints such as fever and weight loss after presumptive exposure to the AIDS virus. These symptoms also occur

13

in the absence of an opportunistic infection and some of these persons may go on to develop the typical manifestations of AIDS.

27. What are the clinical syndromes caused by the AIDS virus?

The original definition of AIDS came about as a tool to better identify and link the individuals who were presenting with unusual infections in the early 1980s. The initial requirements for the diagnosis of AIDS included either an opportunistic infection or Kaposi's sarcoma in the absence of other known causes of immunodeficiency. This definition served well to record the epidemic and develop observations about who was at risk for the illness. It soon became evident, however, that milder conditions related to but clinically distinct from AIDS were appearing in the same populations at risk for AIDS. Once the virus causing AIDS—HIV—was isolated and a blood test to assess exposure was developed, tools were available to suggest that there was a spectrum of HIV-related, transmissible immunodeficiency diseases with AIDS lying at one extreme. The five well-recognized conditions include:

- AIDS
- AIDS-Related Complex (ARC)
- Generalized Lymphadenopathy Syndrome (GLS)
- AIDS virus antibody positivity
- Acute infection

28. How is the AIDS syndrome defined?

The AIDS syndrome was first defined to describe the group of patients who presented with a transmissible immuno-deficiency syndrome in 1981. It was this group who had an opportunistic infection or Kaposi's sarcoma.

29. What is the role of these opportunistic infections?

The majority of the disability in AIDS comes from the opportunistic infections. Autopsies demonstrate that close to 100 percent of persons with AIDS have evidence of at least one opportunistic infection at the time of death. Therefore, given that no specific therapy against either the virus or the immune deficit yet exists, the short-term gains against AIDS will have to come from therapy directed toward the various infections themselves.

30. What are some of these opportunistic infections?

A useful organization to conceptualize the infections is to categorize them into three classes.

First, there are those infections that are responsive to therapy. The organisms causing such infections include the protozoa *Isospora belli*, *Pneumocystis carinii*, and *Toxoplasma gondii*; the fungus *Candida albicans*; and the viruses Herpes simplex and varicella-zoster.

The second group contains those infections for which there is no effective therapy. One organism causing such an infection is the Epstein-Barr virus.

The third classification contains infections caused by those microorganisms for which no conventional therapy exists but for which experimental therapy is currently being evaluated. These include the bacterium *Mycobacterium avium-intracellulare*, cytomegalovirus, and the protozoan Cryptosporidium.

31. Where do these infections occur?

The many infections can be organized by the locations where they occur in the body. The most common infections by organ system are as follows:

Lungs: This is the most commonly involved organ system in AIDS, probably because it represents a wide open portal of entry for all inhaled microorganisms. The lungs are the major target for *Pneumocystis carinii* and are also commonly the site for cytomegalovirus, *Cryptococcus neoformans*, and a variety of typical and atypical tuberculosis bacteria. It is not unusual to see several of these organisms infecting a person with AIDS simultaneously. One infection may be treatable while other coinfecting organisms may be unaffected by whatever drug is given. At autopsy, many persons with AIDS are found to have died from respiratory failure caused either by the lung infection itself or suffered as the result of therapy for the infection.

Skin: This is the preferred site for the cancer Kaposi's sarcoma. The herpes simplex and varicella-zoster viruses can cause painful, deep, and destructive ulcers in many different locations on the skin. The anal region is sometimes affected by the deforming illness known as molluscum contagiosum, another viral disease.

Gastrointestinal: The gastrointestinal tract can be affected anywhere between the lips and the anus. Commonly found microorganisms include herpes simplex virus, which can cause an inflammation of the esophagus (esophagitis), and *Candida albicans*, which causes both oral thrush and esophagitis. Other microorganisms cause intestinal disturbances resulting in debilitating diarrhea and malabsorption of food. These microorganisms include Cryptosporidium, Cytomegalovirus, *Isospora belli*, and *Mycobacterium avium-intracellulare*. Additionally, hairy leukoplakia, a white plaque-like lesion of the tongue associated with several viruses, has also been reported with increased frequency as the initial symptom in persons with AIDS.

Lymph nodes: The nodes can undergo changes from direct infection by organisms such as *Cryptococcus* or tuberculosis bacteria, infiltration by tumor cells of Kaposi's sarcoma, or as the result of infection in the part of the body that is drained by a given node.

Eyes: A small proportion of persons with AIDS have an inflammatory condition of the retina of the eye caused by Cytomegalovirus, which often leads to blindness in the affected eye.

Brain: A majority of persons with AIDS suffer from dramatic changes in the diverse functions of the brain at some time during the course of their disease. Opportunistic infections causing brain disease in persons with AIDS include toxoplasmosis from the protozoan *Toxoplasma gondii*, meningitis from *Cryptococcus neoformans*, and progressive multifocal leukoencephalopathy, a viral illness that slowly erodes the substance of the brain.

It is important to understand that many persons who are not infected with the AIDS virus may at some point in their life develop disease from infection with one of the above microorganisms. This disease may be transient and benign or may run a more fulminant course as the result of factors not related to HIV infection that depress the person's immunity. Presence of such a disease, by itself, does not necessarily imply infection with the AIDS virus and thus does not warrant classifying the person as having an AIDS-related condition. However, evidence of infection with the AIDS virus through blood tests along with the presence of certain opportunistic infection is adequate to classify a particular opportunistic infection as AIDS-related.

32. Is any one of these infections much more common than the others?

The most common opportunistic infection that endangers the life of the person with AIDS is pneumonia caused by *Pneumocystis carinii*. Among AIDS cases reported to the CDC as of February 1987, over 60 percent had been diagnosed with *Pneumocystis carinii*. This pneumonia has an expected mortality rate from 30 to 50 percent for each episode. Drugs do exist to treat this infection; however, 75 percent of AIDS patients will continue to have evidence of what appears to be active disease even after the completion of therapy that is usually curative in non-AIDS patients.

33. Can persons with AIDS minimize the risk of acquiring any of these infections?

Some physicians have recommended that persons with AIDS avoid eating uncooked fish or meat which can contain protozoa and bacteria capable of producing devastating infections in compromised hosts. Cat feces are common sites for *Toxoplasma gondii* and exposure to litter boxes should be avoided. Interaction with other ill persons may result in the development of otherwise preventable infections. Unfortunately, the vast majority of opportunistic infections result from organisms that are widely distributed in nature and are unavoidable.

34. Are there symptoms in persons with AIDS that cannot be explained by opportunistic infections?

Approximately one-third of persons with AIDS have dramatic, deteriorating changes in thinking and consciousness. Manifestations of this condition include headache, disorientation, apathy, memory defects, an inability to concentrate, and alterations in level of consciousness. It currently appears that these changes cannot be attributed solely to the presence of opportunistic brain infections or severe depression, both capable of dramatically altering mental function. Rather, evidence suggests that these changes, in the majority of cases, are the result from the direct effect of the AIDS virus on the brain unrelated to an opportunistic infection. This has been confirmed by the isolation of the virus from cells within the brain and cerebrospinal fluid (CSF) of AIDS patients with neurological symptoms. In addition, AIDS infection has been created in chimpanzees by injecting them with brain tissue from persons with AIDS.

Approximately one-fifth of persons with AIDS have degeneration of the spinal cord that results in neurological symptoms, including severe muscle weakness, difficulty with muscular coordination, and the inability to control urination. As with brain tissue, the AIDS virus has been isolated from spinal cord tissue, suggesting direct infection and involvement of the spinal cord.

Although the original definition of AIDS required the presence of an opportunistic infection or Kaposi's sarcoma coexisting with HIV infection, persons who have HIV-caused neurological symptoms without evidence of an opportunistic infection are now classified as having AIDS. Although these persons can go on to develop an opportunistic infection and thereby resemble the majority of persons with AIDS, why the AIDS virus seems to affect the nervous system preferentially in these persons remains unexplained.

35. Is there any additional significance to the finding that the AIDS virus can infect nervous system cells?

The affinity of the AIDS virus for some cells in the nervous system in addition to helper T-lymphocytes has raised several important issues. A functional barrier exists between the brain's blood vessels and cells that allows some substances from the blood to enter the brain rapidly while preventing other substances from entering at all. This barrier, called the blood-brain barrier, protects the brain from the influence of many substances that rapidly enter other organs from the bloodstream but that are capable of upsetting the delicate function of brain tissue. The likelihood that the brain and spinal cord serve as important locations for the AIDS virus requires that any effective antiviral treatment for AIDS must be able to penetrate the blood-brain barrier.

Researchers have shown that the AIDS virus can be found in the brain within a cell called the macrophage. This cell has important immunological functions such as ingesting foreign substances and serving as a kind of signal to trigger the activation of other cells in the immune system, including the T-lymphocyte. The presence of the virus in macrophages may explain how the blood-brain barrier is overcome in AIDS. Although conclusive studies have not been performed, it is possible that the macrophage rather than the lymphocyte is the cell responsible for carrying the virus from the blood into the tissue of the brain.

It has also been recently observed that the AIDS virus is remarkably similar to visna, a retrovirus with a long incubation period responsible for a slow, progressive neurological disease of sheep. The finding that the AIDS virus has a special affinity for some cells in the nervous system has stimulated interest in retroviruses as possible causative agents of progressive neurological diseases of humans, such as the dementia of Alzheimer's disease.

36. What is known about Kaposi's sarcoma?

Kaposi's sarcoma, a previously rare cancer mainly affecting older men of Mediterranean descent, was included in the original definition of AIDS because of its unusually high frequency in immunocompromised homosexual men, even in the absence of opportunistic infections. This cancer, traditionally sluggish in growth and confined to the skin and lymph nodes, followed a diffuse, destructive course in these immunocompromised individuals. The disease manifests itself clinically as painless purple to brown skin lesions that may be firm or soft, and most often appear on the legs. Later, enlarged lymph nodes develop, suggesting spread of the tumor into the lymphatic system.

As of February 1987, Kaposi's sarcoma had occurred in 24 percent of all persons with AIDS, and is currently the second most common AIDS-associated disease behind *Pneumocystis* pneumonia. While it is unclear why this rare tumor presents itself in AIDS patients, recent work has suggested two possible explanations. While nearly half of homosexual men with AIDS acquire Kaposi's sarcoma, only 4 percent of intravenous drug abusers with AIDS do so, implying that some factor responsible for Kaposi's sarcoma is probably related to sexual contact. Scientific work has isolated fragments of cytomegalovirus in Kaposi tumor cells, suggesting that this virus, capable of being sexually transmitted, may contribute to the development of Kaposi's sarcoma. In addition, preliminary data have shown that the frequency of prior use of "poppers," aerosolized amyl or butyl nitrate reputed to produce an emotional rush during sexual arousal, is greater among those with AIDS and Kaposi's sarcoma compared with those with AIDS and no Kaposi's sarcoma. It may be the case that use of "poppers" during sex and sexual transmission of cytomegalovirus may have a direct, causal effect on the development of Kaposi's sarcoma. Alternately, these factors may be only correlates of other presently unknown factors that result in Kaposi's sarcoma. Although radiotherapy and single drug or combined chemotherapy are presently being explored for the treatment of Kaposi's, most patients usually die of an untreatable infection before completing the course of their treatment.

37. What is the prognosis for persons with AIDS?

As of February 1987, 55 percent of all patients with AIDS reported to the CDC have died. This figure is deceptively low because new cases are being reported at a rate faster than previously. This causes the many new cases to form a higher percentage of all past and present persons with AIDS, tilting the mortality figures to include a disproportionate number of persons early on in the course of their disease, many of whom will go on to die. When one follows a subgroup of persons with AIDS through time, approximately 80 percent will be dead at the end of two years following diagnosis. These figures are especially sobering when one realizes that no person with AIDS has been cured.

38. Are there any factors that influence mortality?

A New York City Department of Health study on over 1,000 persons with AIDS showed that those whose initial symptom was Kaposi's sarcoma alone had an average survival time of 125 weeks. Average survival time dramatically declined to 35 weeks when infection due to *Pneumocystis carinii* was the initial symptom, and was even shorter when persons with combined infections were considered.

39. Can any figures help in appreciating the quality of life of a person with AIDS?

In the same New York City study, 86 percent of all persons with AIDS survived their initial hospitalization. Of these survivors, 46 percent spent approximately one-third of their remaining life in the hospital. Another 32 percent were hospitalized for at least one-half of their remaining days. One must bear in mind that these figures come from the early years of treating the disease. As the number of cases of AIDS increases, as physicians gain more experience with AIDS-related illnesses, and as community resources develop alternatives to hospital settings for medically stable patients, it is likely that the total duration that patients are hospitalized will change.

The diagnosis of AIDS creates personal, social, and psychological crises related to a medical condition that probably have not been experienced to as great a degree since the era of leprosy. Aside from the enormous physical burden a terminal illness places on an individual, it is also clear that the diagnosis of AIDS carries significant psychological costs that defy quantification.

40. When the definition of AIDS was first made, the causative agent was unknown and only individuals with severe opportunistic infections and/or Kaposi's sarcoma were classified as having AIDS. After successfully isolating the

causative virus and after six years of collecting case reports,
has the definition of AIDS been revised to include other
manifestations?

The Conference of State and Territorial Epidemiologists proposed a new definition for AIDS reporting which was recently
approved by the CDC. The definition includes:

- Continued reporting of severe manifestations of opportunistic infections and Kaposi's sarcoma as originally defined.

- In the absence of opportunistic infection, the following
  are indicative of AIDS if the patient has a blood test
  result suggesting prior exposure to the AIDS virus and:

  —widespread histoplasmosis, a fungal disease, not confined only to the lungs or lymph nodes, and diagnosed
  by culture or characteristic microscopic appearance.

  —isosporiasis, a protozoan disease, causing chronic diarrhea for over one month and diagnosed by microscopic appearance of stool or cells.

  —bronchial or pulmonary candidiasis, a fungal disease,
  diagnosed by microscopy or by presence of characteristic lesions seen in the lungs.

  —a specific type of non-Hodgkins's lymphoma, an aggressive tumor of the lymph nodes.

  —Kaposi's sarcoma diagnosed in a patient 60 years of
  age or older at first clinical presentation.

  —chronic lymphoid interstitial pneumonitis, an inflammatory disease of the lung, in a child under 13 years
  of age.

  —a cancer of the lymphatic system diagnosed more than
  three months after the appearance of any opportunistic
  disease.

- Patients will not be included as cases of AIDS if they
  have a negative result on blood testing for exposure to
  the AIDS virus, have no other type of similar test with a
  positive result, and do not have a low number of T-lymphocytes or a low ratio of helper/suppressor T-lymphocytes.

The definition has since been expanded to include those
persons both antibody positive and with neurological disease.

41. What is ARC (AIDS-Related Complex)?

It is possible to view ARC as AIDS without an opportunistic infection or Kaposi's sarcoma. It is a syndrome that is found in those persons who come from risk groups for AIDS, such as homosexual men and intravenous drug abusers. These persons are most often initially seen with weight loss, enlarged lymph nodes, fever, diarrhea, and lethargy. They may also have localized mild infections whose presentation is also seen in persons without severe immunodeficiency. These mild infections include thrush, a fungus-caused disease characterized by white plaques over the surfaces of the inner mouth, and herpes zoster, a viral illness characterized by vesicular, painful, skin eruptions. The notion that ARC is related to the Acquired Immunodeficiency Syndrome comes from the finding of many immune and blood abnormalities, including decreased levels of lymphocytes and other blood cells in these persons. Many of these individuals also demonstrate exposure to the AIDS virus, assessed through blood testing. However, they do not have opportunistic infections and they demonstrate a less severe immunological deficit and clinical course than persons with AIDS. Without either an opportunistic infection or Kaposi's sarcoma characteristic of AIDS, these persons do not meet the CDC definition of having AIDS. In contrast to around 25,000 individuals with AIDS as of December 1986, it is estimated that there are approximately 225,000 persons with ARC.

42. Why not classify persons with ARC as having AIDS? It seems reasonable to argue that persons with ARC have AIDS, just with a less devastating form of the illness.

The distinction among diseases is in many cases arbitrary. Definitions of diseases are constructed in an effort to identify groups of individuals whose history and course of illness are similar enough to allow hypotheses concerning causation, treatment, and prognosis to be tested. It is clear that persons with AIDS differ from those with ARC in at least one major way, the presence of an opportunistic infection. While persons with ARC have been reported to have progressive, terminal courses in some instances, more information on the natural course of these individuals needs to be obtained before the exact relation of ARC to AIDS can be fully understood.

43. Is it possible to make any predictions regarding which persons with ARC will go on to develop AIDS?

A recent study examined 43 persons with ARC and attempted to define factors that would predict which members of this group were at risk for the development of AIDS. During a follow-up period averaging one year, 14, or approximately 30 percent of the group progressed to AIDS. After examining many variables, including prestudy duration of both lymphadenopathy and/or associated symptoms and absolute numbers of T-helper cells, there were two striking factors that predicted the risk of developing AIDS: (1) the nature of symptoms, and (2) the level of gamma interferon, a protein known to play an important role in immune functioning and to be decreased in persons with AIDS.

The 43 persons with ARC were subdivided into four groups: those with lymphadenopathy and (1) herpes zoster, a virally caused skin disease, (2) oral thrush, a fungal disease of the inner mouth characterized by whitish spots, (3) general symptoms such as weight loss, diarrhea, fever, and sore throat, and (4) general symptoms and thrush. Only one of the 15 (7 percent) persons in group one developed AIDS, while the other three groups contained high percentages of persons developing AIDS: $6/14$ or 43 percent of group two, $4/10$ or 40 percent of group three, and ¾ or 75 percent of group four. Most significantly, the levels of gamma interferon were significantly lower for the latter three groups when compared with group one. Indeed, in 9 of the 15 persons with herpes zoster, gamma interferon levels were normal. In contrast, only 2 of the 28 persons in the other three groups, the groups that contained 13 of the 14 persons who developed AIDS, had normal gamma interferon levels. Within each of the three groups with the higher rates of AIDS development, gamma interferon levels were able to differentiate between those who did and did not go on to develop AIDS. While the long-term prognosis for persons with ARC still remains unclear, this study suggests that the risk of developing AIDS one to two years after the diagnosis of ARC may be assessed by correlating symptoms with gamma interferon levels.

Interferon levels are not readily obtained outside of certain research laboratories, and they are not routinely used to assess the likelihood of subsequently developing AIDS once a person has developed ARC. Interferon levels along with other laboratory tests may someday be useful for prognosis purposes, but presently they should be considered investigational tests.

At the present time, persons with ARC number up to ten times the number of persons with AIDS. Consequently, the true risk of developing AIDS after the appearance of ARC in a given patient will not be known until larger prospective studies are performed. Regardless of the risk of developing AIDS from ARC, one must bear in mind that ARC, like AIDS, is a morbid condition that is associated with a significant mortality rate.

44. What is Generalized Lymphadenopathy Syndrome (GLS)?

Concurrent with the initial identification and rapid growth of AIDS cases, an increased incidence of abnormally large lymph nodes, termed generalized lymphadenopathy, was noted in homosexual men and other individuals at high risk for AIDS. This Generalized Lymphadenopathy Syndrome (GLS) is characterized by enlarged lymph nodes with a characteristic pathology of at least three months duration that involves two or more sites outside the groin. These patients do not have opportunistic infections, generalized symptoms such as diarrhea, sore throat, and fever associated with ARC, or other conditions known to decrease immunity. As with ARC, GLS seems to be a condition caused by the AIDS virus leading to a similar underlying defect, yet qualitatively different in symptoms, course, and prognosis.

45. How much is known about the course of individuals with GLS?

Two studies in 1983 and 1985 examined the prognosis of persons diagnosed with GLS. One study followed 90 homosexual men with GLS over a 20-month period. Fifteen of the 90 men developed opportunistic infections, lymphomas, or Kaposi's sarcoma and were reclassified as having AIDS. Of the group of 90 persons, there was a high prevalence of immunological abnormalities, even in those with minimal clinical illness. However, no accurate predictions of which persons, if any, would develop AIDS could be made at the time of initial evaluation. It is also important to note that this study preceded the identification both of the virus causing AIDS and the blood test identifying exposure to it.

The second study followed homosexual men with the benefit of tests to identify prior exposure to the AIDS virus. In this group, 93 men were followed from 3 to 17 months after their diagnosis of GLS. Of these 93 men, 11 developed AIDS. Eighty-five of the men in the study had blood test results showing prior exposure to the AIDS virus, and all 93 had persistent lymphadenopathy. Because these men with GLS also had an epidemiological profile similar to that of persons with AIDS, it is clear that GLS and AIDS are related. The demonstration by a French research team that the same virus isolated from persons with AIDS can be isolated from persons with GLS suggests that GLS is another manifestation of infection with the AIDS virus. Thus, the CDC has included it as a separate category in its listing of the various clinical forms of infection with the AIDS virus. However, it remains to be seen whether the lymphadenopathy characteristic of this condition is an inevitable precursor to AIDS or whether it represents a distinct illness that may progress to AIDS in only some cases.

46. What is the condition represented by "AIDS virus antibody positivity"?

A blood test reflecting prior exposure to and infection with the AIDS virus has been developed. This test detects the antibodies that are produced after infection with the AIDS virus. A significant number of individuals in high risk AIDS groups such as homosexual men and intravenous drug users have been shown to have antibody to the AIDS virus, suggesting prior exposure. Because retroviral infections are likely to be lifelong, prior exposure is considered by many scientists to be equivalent to current infection. However, an individual with antibody positivity, also termed seropositivity, is not synonymous with that person having AIDS or any of its other clinical manifestations. In fact, the majority of persons with antibody positive results are asymptomatic. These antibody positive persons are able to transmit the virus to others and thereby serve as unknowing participants in the spread of the virus into increasingly larger numbers of people. It is estimated that there are from 1 to 1.5 million Americans who are infected with the AIDS virus and are antibody positive.

47. What is meant by the condition of "acute infection"?

An acute flu-like illness characterized by fever, enlarged lymph nodes, malaise, skin rash, sore muscles, and diarrhea has been described in some individuals within three to six weeks after exposure to the AIDS virus through sexual contact, blood transfusion, or intravenous drug use. The condition, which resolves quickly, is considered to be an initial reaction to infection with the AIDS virus. This acute infection has been documented in several persons by virus isolation during the acute illness and by the finding of concurrent or subsequent conversion to AIDS antibody positivity. The recent finding of transient neurological dysfunction, including disorientation and seizures associated with the conversion to antibody positivity in two individuals adds these symptoms to the already well-described clinical correlates of acute AIDS virus infection.

While many persons with AIDS retrospectively report these transient symptoms, other persons have been identified as having this acute infection and not progressing to AIDS. The significance of these symptoms will become clearer as individuals are followed from the point that they first become ill and data concerning their immunological function and symptoms are collected.

48. What evidence clarifies how these syndromes are precursors of AIDS?

A San Francisco clinic study retrospectively reviewed blood collected in the late 1970s from 6,875 homosexual men. By 1980, 1,684 or 24.5 percent of these men were antibody positive, 2 had developed AIDS, and the ratio of antibody positive-to-AIDS cases in this group was 825:1 [1,684:2]. When retested in 1985, the number of men with antibody positive findings had increased to 5,053 or 74 percent of the original sample. By this time, 202 or 3 percent of all the men in the original group had developed AIDS. Thus, the antibody positivity-to-AIDS case ratio in these men had dropped from 825:1 in 1980 to about 25:1 in 1985. It is from this type of data that the number of antibody positive-to-AIDS cases in the general population at any given time has been estimated at about 100:1. This does not imply that only 1 of 100 infected individuals will go on to develop AIDS but instead reflects an estimate of the total number of antibody positive persons-to-AIDS cases at a single point in time.

When groups of people with antibody positive findings are followed through time, a significant percentage of these persons go on to develop AIDS or an AIDS-related illness. For example, 31 individuals in the aforementioned study who were antibody positive from 1978 to 1980 were recontacted and allowed investigators to follow their health over a median time of about 5 years: two (7 percent) developed the AIDS syndrome, and eight others (26 percent) developed ARC, GLS, or blood abnormalities. Additional studies following infected homosexual men over a period of years have found similar results: approximately 20 to 25 percent develop AIDS-related conditions such as ARC and GLS within five years of infection, while approximately 10 percent develop AIDS in that period. Once again, it is important to note that these data involved the study of homosexual men and may not be generalizable to other groups.

49. What is the interval between AIDS virus infection and the onset of AIDS symptoms?

Three to six weeks after infection is the time period when most persons exhibit the transient symptoms associated with acute infection. The average time between infection and appearance of symptoms of AIDS, termed the incubation period of the AIDS virus, is estimated to be about three years. This estimate is based on retrospective reviews of single transfusion-associated cases. Because AIDS was initially recognized as a syndrome only as recently as 1981, those cases with a longer incubation period may have not yet occurred. The shortest incubation period for AIDS or a related illness has been the occurrence of ARC in a man seven weeks after receiving a contaminated blood transfusion.

50. What is the most current CDC classification of AIDS-related conditions?

In mid-1986, the CDC published a reclassification of the various manifestations of HIV infection to understand more fully the scope of the disease and incorporate prior redefinitions of AIDS. This classification scheme was intended to allow better health care planning, improve public health control strategies, and provide more comprehensive epidemiological data and optimal patient care. This classification system is such that persons can only be classified into more advanced groups as their symptoms and signs change and, consistent with the definition of having an AIDS-related condition, all persons must have antibody positive findings for the AIDS virus.

Group 1	Acute infection
Group 2	Asymptomatic infection (antibody positivity)
Group 3	Persistent Generalized Lymphadenopathy Syndrome (GLS)
Group 4	Other disease
Subgroup A	Constitutional disease (ARC)
Subgroup B	Neurological disease (AIDS)
Subgroup C	Infectious diseases (AIDS)
Subgroup C-1	Specific infectious diseases listed in the CDC definition of AIDS (see Question 40)
Subgroup C-2	Other specified infectious diseases (such as tuberculosis, hairy leukoplakia, and herpes zoster)
Subgroup D	Specified Cancers (such as Kaposi's sarcoma) (AIDS)
Subgroup E	Other immunological conditions influenced by HIV infection.

CHAPTER THREE

Who Gets AIDS?
Groups at Risk

51. The definition of AIDS, what causes it, many of the symptoms, and some related immunodeficiency conditions in high risk groups have been mentioned. What types of people get AIDS, what constitutes a high risk group, and does this tell us anything new about the modes of transmissibility?

As of May 1, 1987, 35,219 cases of AIDS had been reported to the CDC. Of these, 34,725 were adults and 494 were children 13 years of age or younger. The breakdown of groups was as follows:

Adults

73 percent: homosexual or bisexual men*

17 percent: heterosexual users of intravenous drugs from dirty (nonsterile) needles

 4 percent: heterosexual male or female partners of persons with AIDS or at risk for acquiring AIDS†

---

*Eight percent of these males also reported a history of intravenous drug abuse.

†This group is composed of 51 percent males and 49 percent females; in addition, 53 percent were born in countries outside the United States where heterosexual transmission is thought to be the primary means of acquiring AIDS.

3 percent: unable or yet to be classified into any known
             risk group‡
2 percent: received a blood transfusion within five years
             preceding onset of their illness
1 percent: hemophiliacs receiving blood products

Children and Infants

80 percent: born to parent with AIDS or at increased risk for
             acquiring AIDS
12 percent: transfusion related
5 percent: hemophiliac related
3 percent: unable or yet to be classified into any known
             risk group

---

‡This group consists of persons for whom risk information was unavailable
secondary to death of the patient, refusal to be interviewed, inability to
locate the patient, men whose only risk factor was contact with a prostitute
whose antibody status was unknown, those currently under investigation,
and those in whom no risk factor could be identified.

CHAPTER FOUR

How AIDS Is Acquired: Modes of Transmissibility

52. *Why did AIDS first appear principally in male homosexuals in the United States?*

The homosexual connection with AIDS has been both distorted and misinterpreted. While it is clear that male homosexuals represent the group with the largest percentage of all cases of AIDS reported to date in the United States, a careful analysis has revealed the special characteristics of the homosexual population that led to this misfortune. The association between AIDS and homosexuals was first noted in reports of the several hundred earliest cases of AIDS. Although a variety of explanations was proposed to explain the sudden appearance of this syndrome in homosexual men, when homosexual men with and without AIDS were compared the only clearly distinguishing feature between the two groups was the average number of sexual partners during the preceding year. The men with AIDS averaged 61 sex partners in the preceding year compared with 25 partners for the healthy group over the same time period.

When the virus causing AIDS was identified, the homosexual connection with AIDS became better understood. Any small group that has sexual contacts principally limited to the members of that group has amplified chances of spreading a sexually transmissible disease among its members. If, for example, another defined subpopulation had a higher prevalence of the transmissible virus among its members but these persons were monogamous, then the virus would not spread beyond those initially infected. It is not surprising, therefore, that many of the first homosexuals with AIDS identified in the United States had over 1,000 sex partners in their lifetime.

This degree of sexual activity markedly increased their chance of meeting an individual carrying the virus at a time when it was relatively rare. As AIDS is a disease that is capable of being transmitted through sexual contact, the incidence in a given population is proportional, as with all venereal diseases, to the number of sexual contacts. The principal reason for the higher incidence of AIDS in the male homosexual population was its early appearance in this group followed by its spread through a high level of sexual activity in a sexually self-contained group.

53. How is the virus sexually spread among homosexuals?

Male homosexuals engage in a variety of sex practices, several of which result in exposure to feces, blood, and semen. These bodily fluids may be introduced through oral, genital, or rectal routes. It is nearly impossible to weigh the relative risk of each sex practice since a given homosexual with AIDS will be likely to have had a number of different partners and to have engaged in different sexual practices. Clearly, contact with blood and semen are felt to be the major routes involved in transmission of the AIDS virus.

54. How do blood and semen transmit the virus?

Both blood and semen carry the virus in infected persons. To develop AIDS, it is thought that the virus must make its way into the bloodstream and infect lymphocytes. Infected blood or semen can presumably find its way through small breaks in the linings of the mouth, rectum, and perhaps even through skin. The finding that artificial insemination has resulted in the development of GLS in a woman with no prior risk factor for AIDS is further demonstration that semen can transmit the virus with minimal trauma in a single exposure.

55. Can the AIDS virus be transmitted through oral sex?

It seems possible given the nature of the exposure. No person with AIDS has been reported as engaging solely in this sex act apart from other sexual practices, making ideal assessment of this question difficult. However, a similarity between oral and rectal intercourse is exposure to semen. While speculative, it may be that the virus can make its way through small or even microscopic breaks in the lining of the mouth to the bloodstream where it can infect T-lymphocytes.

56. How is rectal intercourse implicated in the transmission of the virus?

This sex practice is highly suspected as a means of transmitting the virus. Rectal intercourse often leads to breaks in the lining of the rectum which can serve as a portal of entry for the virus from the semen. Homosexuals with AIDS routinely report high levels of genital-anal sex. Antibody prevalence studies show that in homosexual men practicing anal intercourse, the insertive partner has a slightly lower chance of developing antibodies to the AIDS virus than the receptive partner. Both activities, however, are associated with transmission of the AIDS virus.

57. Lesbians are homosexuals. Do they also get AIDS?

AIDS is not prevalent among lesbians as a group. Naturally, a lesbian is as susceptible as any individual given a "critical exposure," that is, exposure to another infected person through any known means of AIDS virus transmission.

58. Does that mean that heterosexuals have just as much likelihood as homosexuals of contracting the AIDS virus if they have a critical sexual exposure?

Yes. Because the AIDS virus is spread through semen and blood, any sexual activity that involves exposure to infected semen or blood is potentially capable of spreading the virus. The case for heterosexual activity with multiple partners as a risk factor for AIDS virus transmission is supported most strongly by evidence from Central Africa. There, AIDS is known to affect women as frequently as men, and is highly associated with a large subpopulation of female prostitutes and the men who are their sexual contacts.

Many people have the mistaken belief that some aspect of homosexuality per se is responsible for AIDS. In fact, any person engaging in sexual contact outside of a monogamous relationship potentially exposes himself to all the partners with whom the new sex partner has been in contact. With one new sex partner, one could conceivably expose oneself to the cumulative risks of thousands of contacts never intended to be met. This partner could be homosexual, heterosexual, male, female, symptomatic, or asymptomatic for AIDS.

One can imagine other groups besides homosexuals with a greater-than-average number of sexual contacts. Sex between many individuals and a prostitute, sexual contacts between prisoners when the special circumstances of incarceration often lead to multiple homosexual encounters, or any contact between an individual and a commonly shared sexual partner are all examples of subgroups in which the AIDS virus could have been propagated with reasonable success. AIDS arrived in the homosexual population first because of some random encounter with the virus. Subgroups with high sexual activity may still have to contend with the virus at a later date as it increases its spread through the heterosexual population.

59. Have any of these special situations been encountered?

Male prisoners constitute a special subgroup of those with a higher-than-average prevalence of AIDS. As of early 1986, 766 cases of AIDS had been reported among inmates of all 50 state correctional institutions, 37 large city and county jails, and all federal prisons. Intravenous drug abuse or homosexual activity appeared to be the means of AIDS transmission in most of these inmates.

As a result of this rate of AIDS among prisoners, different prisons and jails have instituted various policies for their inmates. For example, over 80 percent of correctional facilities now provide educational materials on AIDS to staff and inmates. Testing for exposure to the AIDS virus is mandatory for all incoming inmates in 6 state prisons and 7 city or county jails, while 39 state prisons and 20 city/county jails test for such exposure only when inmates appear to be in high risk groups or when clinically warranted. Housing policies regarding segregation of inmates with AIDS or infection also vary between facilities. For example, while allowing healthy but infected inmates to remain in the general prison population, state prisons in Florida, New Jersey, and New York, as well as New York City jails, medically isolate those prisoners with AIDS. Eight state prisons and 13 city/county jails, on the other hand, have adopted policies that require segregation of all infected inmates to hospitals, housing units, or cells.

60. What is the mechanism for heterosexual female-to-male transmission?

It is well recognized that female-to-male sexual transmission of the AIDS virus can occur. There are a number of possible mechanisms for this transmission: (1) the virus has recently been isolated from the vaginal and/or cervical secretions of four of eight women with antibody positive findings, albeit in amounts less than that usually found in infected blood and semen, (2) the isolation of infectious virus from saliva, also in smaller concentrations than that found in infected blood and semen, raises the additional possibility of spread of the virus through intimate salivary exchange, and (3) menstrual blood may also figure in the transmission of the virus.

61. What role do female prostitutes have in the transmission of AIDS?

Studies of female prostitutes have helped to demonstrate that heterosexual female-to-male transmission of the AIDS virus occurs. Many studies show a high prevalence of antibody positivity in prostitutes both in the United States and Africa. One study in Central Africa found 29 of 33 randomly studied prostitutes were antibody positive. Of these 33 prostitutes, 26 had symptoms related to AIDS. Of male customers in that same area, the incidence of antibody positivity rose rapidly with increasing numbers of sexual contacts. In East Africa, over half of 90 female prostitutes studied were antibody positive, and GLS was present in 54 percent of these antibody positive prostitutes. In both the United States and Africa, a large number of men categorized into "no known risk group" have reported frequent contacts with female prostitutes.

The recent estimate that approximately one-third of all women entering treatment for narcotic addiction in the United States have at one time engaged in prostitution suggests that some prostitutes have an added high risk means of being exposed to the AIDS virus. Contact with prostitutes may serve as a bridge between high risk groups and low risk heterosexual customers. These customers may further propagate the virus into the general population, thereby leading to an increasing incidence of AIDS in heterosexuals.

Because the majority of AIDS cases in the United States has occurred in homosexual men, the emphasis has been on male-to-male and male-to-female virus transmission. The increasing number of infected heterosexual men without prior risk factors who report contact with female prostitutes has increased attention on female-to-male transmission of the AIDS virus.

62. What is the percentage of AIDS cases in the United States thought to be the result of heterosexual contact?

Among the 34,725 adult cases of AIDS reported to CDC as of May 1, 1987, approximately 68 percent were thought to be related to sexual contact. Approximately 4 percent of the total number of AIDS cases were in heterosexual individuals who were not intravenous drug abusers and did not fit into other known risk categories such as sexual contact with homosexual men, receiving a blood transfusion, or being a hemophiliac.

63. Does the homosexual population in the United States figure in the transmission of AIDS virus elsewhere?

It is probable that in many cases the AIDS virus was transmitted from American male homosexuals to their European partners. While homosexual/bisexual men make up 73 percent of United States cases, approximately 50 percent of all European cases involve homosexual men. Of the affected European homosexual men, 75 percent have reported sexual contact with an American homosexual preceding the onset of their illness. The earlier identification of AIDS in the United States, the greater number of affected persons, and the aforementioned data strongly suggest that AIDS was probably spread in large numbers from the United States to Europe.

64. In the breakdown of who gets AIDS, it is mentioned that persons have acquired AIDS from someone "at risk" for the disease. What does "at risk" refer to?

At risk individuals have previously engaged in behaviors at high risk for AIDS virus transmission. They are usually healthy, antibody positive, carry the virus, and are capable of infecting others. The AIDS virus has, in fact, been isolated from the blood of many of these healthy, antibody positive individuals. Although one certainly does not have to be in a recognized risk group such as intravenous drug abusers or homosexual men to have antibody positive results, the majority of at risk persons do come from groups who engage in behaviors that increase their likelihood of contracting the virus and acting as a carrier. The ability of a healthy person to act as a carrier who can transmit the AIDS virus to others receives further support from the presence of antibodies to the AIDS virus in asymptomatic mothers whose offspring develop AIDS.

65. What about intravenous drug abusers?

About one-fifth of all cases of AIDS in the United States occur in intravenous drug abusers, a larger figure than occurs in Europe. The mode of AIDS transmission is the use of nonsterile needles in nonmedical settings which transmits the virus from the blood of one individual to another. In this group, men predominate over women about 4:1. The New York-New Jersey area has provided the bulk of these cases, with only about 15 percent coming from outside of that region.

The presentation of AIDS in this group is quite different from that in the homosexual population because of the infrequent appearance of Kaposi's sarcoma. As mentioned earlier, Kaposi's sarcoma occurs frequently in populations in which sexual transmission is the primary mode of acquiring AIDS. In intravenous drug users who contract AIDS, *Pneumocystis carinii* and other opportunistic infections represent the more typical initial clinical presentation.

66. Do intravenous drug abusers have any other special role in the propagation of AIDS?

It appears that intravenous drug abusers are a major connection in the transmission of the AIDS virus among heterosexuals and from the homosexual-to-heterosexual population. A recent study in the New York area examined the drug use patterns and the sexual habits of a group of intravenous drug abusers. These individuals were composed of those with AIDS, ARC, and no apparent disease (although serological status was not mentioned). Of the 40 persons with AIDS or ARC, 88 percent admitted to sharing needles routinely. Furthermore, 74 percent of the original 40 individuals admitted to attending "shooting galleries" where needles are passed widely among many anonymous individuals also injecting drugs. In addition, approximately half of the persons with AIDS admitted to sharing needles with either known or suspected homosexuals. This suggests a likely continuous introduction of the virus from the homosexual population to the population of intravenous drug users, the majority of whom are heterosexual. The clear link between these two groups demonstrates that needle sharing among intravenous drug abusers will probably remain a vital means of introducing the AIDS virus into the heterosexual population.

Approximately 8 percent of homosexual and bisexual men with AIDS report intravenous drug abuse. Estimates also indicate that in some cities from 60 to 90 percent of intravenous drug abusers, heterosexual and homosexual, are antibody positive. With these numbers in mind, it seems reasonable to postulate that intravenous drug abuse represents an important link between these currently well-circumscribed risk groups and the population at large.

67. In what ways do children with AIDS differ from adults with AIDS?

The virus can be transmitted to children in ways similar to adults. However, the majority of children with AIDS or AIDS virus infection are thought to have been exposed to the virus while in the uterus of or during delivery by a mother who either had AIDS, appeared healthy but was in a high risk group for AIDS, or was the sexual partner of someone in a high risk group. Of the approximately 350 cases of children with AIDS, about 50 percent had mothers who were intravenous drug abusers, 17 percent had mothers who were born in Haiti, and 10 percent had mothers who were sex partners of either intravenous drug abusers or bisexual men. In addition to AIDS, AIDS virus infection in children can also lead to ARC and asymptomatic infection.

Recognition of AIDS virus transmission during pregnancy, labor, or delivery rather than during the period after birth has been strongly supported by two AIDS cases occurring in children who had no contact with their infected mothers after birth. In addition, the isolation of the AIDS virus from a 20-week old aborted fetus of an antibody positive intravenous drug abuser is further evidence of the intrauterine transmission of the AIDS virus. The mode of transmission from mother to fetus is assumed to be virus passage across the placenta.

In contrast to adults, the average time between exposure to the virus and onset of symptoms is four months in children with AIDS. Children with AIDS, however, suffer from similar infections and have the same dismal prognosis as adults with AIDS.

68. Do infants infected with the AIDS virus in utero have any unusual physical features that can distinguish them at birth?

Intrauterine infection with the AIDS virus has recently been shown to be capable of causing serious abnormalities in fetal development. When 20 infants and children with AIDS or ARC were examined, the following abnormal features were present: (1) growth failure (97 percent of all healthy children the same age showed greater height and weight), (2) a small head (97 percent of all children the same age had a bigger head circumference), and (3) an unusual physical appearance, including a prominent forehead, short nose with a flattened bridge, prominent upper lip, and an atypical appearance of the eyes. Each of these features occurred in 50 to 75 percent of the children, and collectively were thought to represent a new syndrome related to intrauterine AIDS infection and to be distinct from other acquired birth defects. Most importantly, appearance of these features in infants may be the first indication of infection with the AIDS virus, thereby necessitating further medical evaluation.

69. Can infected mothers safely breast-feed their infants?

A case has been reported where AIDS developed in a breast-fed baby whose previously unexposed mother acquired the virus through a blood transfusion after the birth of her child. Recently, the AIDS virus has been isolated from the breast milk of infected women. It seems, therefore, that breast feeding may be another mode of transmission of the virus from mother to infant, although children have been breast-fed by antibody positive mothers without developing the antibodies to the AIDS virus.

70. Can children infected with the AIDS virus be vaccinated for other infectious diseases, similar to what is done in uninfected children?

Children routinely receive vaccinations for a variety of infectious diseases while they are young. These vaccinations involve administering an inactive or attenuated microorganism whose introduction into the body typically evokes an immune response without producing disease. Although the vast majority of children have no difficulty with the treatments and go on to make antibodies against the intended organism, a small number of children do have adverse reactions after vaccination.

Some of the children who respond atypically to the vaccine are immunosuppressed before vaccination for reasons unrelated to AIDS. As a result, many physicians are concerned about the risk of introducing certain microorganisms through vaccination into children already infected with the AIDS virus who are potentially immunosuppressed. This decrease in immunity, in turn, could make the children more susceptible to the adverse effects of vaccines that employ attenuated viruses. To address this concern, the CDC published guidelines in early 1987 for immunization practices in children.

Just as in adults, children infected with the AIDS virus can be divided into two large groups—those who are infected but have no evidence of illness, and those who are infected and who do have clinical evidence of illness. The CDC recommended unchanged vaccination practices for asymptomatic children with one minor exception. The bulk of children who are infected with the AIDS virus come from homes where the adults are members of other high risk groups. Consequently, the CDC advised caution with these children in the use of attenuated vaccines, such as the oral polio vaccine. This caution is advised not because of the risk of disease to the child being vaccinated but to address the theoretical risk of spreading disease to the unvaccinated, immunosuppressed adults who are cohabitating in the home. This scenario remains hypothetical as no reports of infection with vaccine microorganisms in antibody positive household contacts of vaccinated children have occurred.

For those children who are infected with the AIDS virus and who show clinical signs of illness related to the AIDS virus, there are changes in the standard recommendations. The use of any attenuated vaccine, such as the oral polio vaccine, the mumps, measles, and rubella vaccine, or the tuberculosis vaccine is not advised. Because adverse effects have not been seen in children when immunized with vaccines that employ inactivated organisms, routine vaccinations that use inactivated organisms should continue as in normal circumstances.

Because children infected with the AIDS virus often have significant immunological abnormalities, vaccinations not normally used in children with normal immunity were suggested to help prevent the occurrence of other disease. The CDC recommended the use of inactivated influenza vaccine on an annual basis, coupled with a one-time use of the pneumococcal vaccine. After known exposures to measles or varicella (chicken pox), the committee advised the use of immune globulin to prevent the occurrence of those infections.

71. Has any child contracted AIDS from another child?

Unlike adults, sharing of dirty needles and sexual contact have not been significant means of virus transmission in this group. Like adults, there is no evidence that the transmission of AIDS virus can occur through casual contact. Thus, there is no known case of a child acquiring AIDS through school, day care, or foster care settings through typical contact with another child.

72. Define casual contact.

Casual contact includes touching, holding, living in the same house as a person with AIDS, breathing the same air as a person with AIDS, being coughed upon or eating food prepared by an infected person, or any other activity that does not involve exposure of the blood, saliva, or semen of an infected person to the blood or mucous membranes of another. Aside from the lack of evidence to indicate transmission of the virus through any of these means, there is also no evidence that the AIDS virus can be transmitted through the use of swimming pools, spas, hot tubs, or toilets previously used by an infected individual.

Studies of nonsexual household contacts of persons with AIDS strengthen the belief that casual contact with saliva does not result in transmission of the virus. For example, a recent study examined 101 family members who had shared a household and most of the above activities with a person with AIDS but who were not sexual partners of the person. Excluding one child believed to have acquired the infection before birth, no evidence of antibody positive results, abnormal T-lymphocyte profiles, or the presence of AIDS was found in these individuals an average of three years after initial exposure to their infected family members. It is also noteworthy that no cases of AIDS related to casual contact have been found in health care workers intimately involved in the care of AIDS patients.

73. Doesn't the isolation of the AIDS virus from saliva imply the possible transmission through casual contact such as kissing?

The isolation of the AIDS virus from saliva has raised questions and confusion about possible casual transmission of the

AIDS virus despite no reported cases of such transmission. The finding that the AIDS virus was isolated from only 1 of 83 saliva samples from 71 infected men suggests that the AIDS virus is found infrequently in the saliva of infected persons. In the one sample from which the virus was isolated, the level of virus present was low and much lower than that found in the blood. This supports the lack of antibody positive results and AIDS reported from household members and health care workers exposed to the saliva of persons with AIDS. Despite an absence of cases showing infection from casual contact such as kissing, the poorly understood mechanism of female-to-male transmission of the AIDS virus and the demonstration that the virus can survive at room temperature outside of the body for up to 15 days supports the continued practice of careful hygiene around those with AIDS.

74. Doesn't the presence of a group without known risk factors imply the possibility of transmission of AIDS virus through casual contact?

No. Again, there are no cases of AIDS or AIDS virus infection that have been identified as resulting from transmission of the AIDS virus through casual contact. This includes not only evaluation of the casual contacts of thousands of persons with AIDS but also the evaluation of thousands of health care workers who have antibody negative results after casual contact with those having AIDS virus infection.

Those persons with AIDS who are categorized by the CDC into the group without known risk factors include those who could not be interviewed prior to their death, those who refused to be interviewed, those who had known sexual contacts with prostitutes but where the antibody status of the prostitute was unknown, and those whose risk factors were still under investigation at the time of their classification.

Nearly 75 percent of those with AIDS who were initially classified as having no known risk factors were later reclassified after additional investigation. This fact further supports the notion that the number of those with AIDS and no known risk factors is probably much smaller than 3 percent of total AIDS cases reported to the CDC.

75. What is a hemophiliac?

Hemophiliacs are born with an inherited bleeding disorder and are usually male. This disorder is genetically determined and results in poor blood clotting because of the absence of a single protein involved with coagulation. In the past, hemophiliacs faced a markedly shortened life filled with a multitude of bleeding complications. That dismal prognosis changed with the introduction of a concentrated clotting factor. Clotting factor is derived from the blood of between 2,500 to 25,000 donors. By injecting the clotting factor, a hemophiliac can approach having what is considered to be normal clotting of the blood.

76. How do hemophiliacs fit into the AIDS picture?

As cases of AIDS began to accumulate, it became clear that one of the principal groups at risk were hemophiliacs who were neither users of intravenous drugs nor homosexual. The link between the other risk groups and hemophiliacs was the hemophiliac's repeated exposure to derivatives of human blood potentially contaminated with the AIDS virus. The apparent implication that hemophiliacs were at risk solely because of their use of clotting factor suggested that AIDS could appear outside of groups physically contacting one another. Even before the virus causing AIDS was isolated, the hemophiliac experience strongly suggested, as in the case of drug abusers, that AIDS was probably spread by a transmissible agent. Until screening for the virus became possible and widely used, hemophiliacs were exposed to the cumulative risks of many thousands of people with each new vial of clotting factor.

77. Can hemophiliacs substitute something for clotting factor?

A smaller number of blood donors supply the blood that goes into the preparation of cryoprecipitate, an alternative to clotting factor. It is a blood product with less of the necessary clotting factors for hemophiliacs and can be used with some success in hemophiliacs who have not totally lost their ability to clot blood. While initial reports indicate fewer immunological abnormalities in hemophiliacs receiving cryoprecipitate, there are cases of AIDS in those who have received only this preparation.

78. Do all hemophiliacs run similar risks for HIV infection?

There are different forms of hemophilia. Those with hemophilia A have hereditary low levels of the protein factor VIII. When they have a nearly total absence of the clotting factor, they are classified as severe hemophiliacs. Others have less severe disease but still need additional factor VIII to clot properly. The CDC noted in May 1985 that the severely affected group continued to constitute approximately 70 percent of all AIDS cases noted in hemophiliacs. The less severe hemophiliacs who need less factor VIII and are able to use cryoprecipitate, comprised about 13 percent. The remainder of the cases of AIDS in hemophiliacs came from the other forms of hemophilia, specifically von Willebrand's disease, hemophilia B (hereditary factor IX deficiency), and acquired inhibitors to the clotting proteins.

The original preponderance of cases detected in the severely affected type A hemophiliacs has proportionately decreased while the less severely affected hemophiliacs have begun to account for a higher percentage of newly reported cases. Exposure to the virus in the severely affected hemophiliacs resulted from the need for more clotting factor. The less severely affected hemophiliacs needed fewer blood products and encountered smaller donor pools through the use of cryoprecipitate. However, with increasing time these lower risk hemophiliacs were exposed to infected blood products and now comprise an increasingly larger proportion of hemophiliacs contracting AIDS. The implication is clear; the virus could be passed through either form of clotting factor preparation and expose hemophiliacs to the risk of acquiring AIDS.

79. What is the risk to a hemophiliac of getting AIDS?

As with most of the risk groups for AIDS, the data are still accumulating. More definitive information will be known after years of careful follow up of infected hemophiliacs. Preliminary data reported by the CDC in late 1984 showed that of over 200 hemophiliacs surveyed, 74 percent of type A hemophiliacs and 39 percent of type B hemophiliacs had positive results for the AIDS antibody. In some centers, the rate of antibody positivity in those with severe hemophilia A approaches 95 percent.

Estimates emphasizing the very high risk of prior exposure to the AIDS virus for hemophiliacs have been made. As of early 1986, there were approximately 70 hemophiliacs with AIDS in the United States. Among these patients, earlier studies had shown that they had not used any common vials of clotting factor. Thus, if one reasonably assumes that each of the 70 different hemophiliacs obtained his clotting factor from a different pool that was distributed among 100 hemophiliacs, then approximately 7,000 of the 10,000 hemophiliacs in the United States have been exposed to the AIDS virus. While the number of AIDS cases made up of hemophiliacs is small in comparison to the other risk groups, more hemophiliac cases of AIDS should be expected as more of those previously infected become symptomatic.

80. What is being done about the risk of AIDS in hemophiliacs?

In 1984 the Medical and Scientific Advisory Council of the National Hemophilia Foundation provided new guidelines for the therapy of hemophilia. They advised that (1) cryoprecipitate be used in children under four, in infants with factor VIII deficiency, and in newly diagnosed hemophiliacs with factor VIII deficiency, (2) fresh frozen plasma, a solution containing clotting proteins, should be used for the preceding groups when a factor IX deficiency is present, and (3) DDAVP, another blood product that improves clotting, should be used when possible as an alternative to factor VIII concentrate in those with mild cases of factor VIII deficiency.

Experiments that introduce the AIDS virus into factor VIII concentrate and then subject it to high temperature have shown that the level of the virus can be dramatically reduced with short periods of treatment. If the heat treatment process is continued for a minimum of 24 hours, the virus can no longer be detected. Consequently, the National Hemophilia Foundation has recommended the use of heat-treated factor VIII concentrate in place of the routine factor VIII preparation. Data from Europe already suggest that chidren exposed only to heat-treated factor VIII are less likely to become antibody positive when compared with children who are exposed to factor VIII without heat treatment. In addition, preliminary data suggest that treatment of infected blood with certain chemicals (such as 0.3% tri(n-butyl)phosphate (TNBP/0.2% sodium cholate [CA]) also appears to inactivate the AIDS virus while leaving clotting factors unaffected. This finding holds great promise for the wide-scale use of chemically treated factor VIII concentrate in hemophiliacs but careful observation of those given this concentrate is necessary before its effectiveness and safety can be confirmed.

The fact that AIDS may exceed bleeding as the leading cause of death in hemophiliacs highlights the significance of AIDS to this group. The continued development of chemicals and procedures that inactivate the AIDS virus while leaving clotting factor unaffected, the avoidance of high risk persons as blood donors, and the use of the AIDS antibody screening test to identify blood that comes from virus-exposed individuals are necessary if hemophiliacs are to avoid exposure to the virus through their injections of clotting factors.

81. Hepatitis B vaccine is made from human blood products. Is there a risk of catching AIDS from hepatitis B vaccine?

No cases of an association between hepatitis B vaccine and AIDS have been documented. The vaccine has been undergoing tests of efficacy since the late 1970s. Since identification of the AIDS virus, three inactivation steps used to prepare the vaccine (treatment with formalin, urea, and pepsin) have been shown to reduce the AIDS virus to undetectable levels in known contaminated samples. These inactivation procedures are routinely used in hepatitis B vaccine preparation and inactivate all known animal viruses.

82. Often, individuals receive pooled immunoglobulin injections as protection to minimize the risk of acquiring some viral diseases following an exposure. Is this product safe to receive?

There have been no cases of AIDS attributed to the use of pooled immunoglobulin proteins. This product is collected antibodies from hundreds of blood donors and is often used to protect against hepatitis after an exposure. Review of the procedure used in preparation of the immunoglobulins suggests that the routine treatment with ethyl alcohol probably inactivates the virus.

83. If AIDS has been shown to be transmissible in protein preparations from blood and blood products, are there any other ways one might be unknowingly exposed to AIDS through products utilizing such proteins?

The CDC reported in 1985 that a private clinic in the Bahamas had been offering cancer patients vials of human serum protein unapproved for use in the United States. This unproven cancer treatment, termed immunoaugmentive therapy, purportedly restores immune functioning by injection of proteins derived from tumor tissue and blood from large numbers of patients and volunteers. In May 1985, two separate United States laboratories tested samples of these proteins supplied by two patients. Eight of the 18 samples were either repeatedly antibody positive or borderline positive. Subsequently, the CDC was able to isolate viable AIDS virus from one of these samples. In July 1985, the clinic closed.

84. Summarize the ways AIDS can be transmitted through blood.

Individuals who have used dirty, nonsterile needles to administer street drugs, those who have received contaminated blood transfusions or blood products, and children who develop AIDS from an infected mother *in utero* or at birth are examples of persons whose AIDS transmission is thought to occur through blood-borne routes.

85. Who should refrain from donating blood?

The CDC advises individuals in the following risk groups to avoid blood donation: persons with clinical or laboratory evidence of HIV infection, men who have had sex with another man one or more times since 1977, current or past intravenous drug abusers, persons emigrating since 1977 from countries where heterosexual activity is thought to play a major role in transmission of HIV (such as Haiti and countries in Central Africa), persons with hemophilia who have received clotting factor concentrates, sexual partners of any persons in the above categories, men and women who have engaged in prostitution since 1977, and persons who have been heterosexual partners of prostitutes within six months of a prospective donation.

86. If AIDS can be transmitted through blood, should blood be donated to blood bank centers?

Yes, if you are not in one of the groups who should refrain from donating. As in all medically supervised settings, needles used for individuals donating blood are sterile, previously unused, and disposed of immediately after use. Therefore, under these conditions, donating blood provides zero risk of contracting AIDS. During the first few weeks of January 1986, the American Association of Blood Banks reported a severe nationwide shortage in blood supply, presumably related to the unfounded fear by many of acquiring AIDS through blood donation.

87. Risk groups in which semen and blood are the recognized routes of AIDS virus transmission have been mentioned. But, the breakdown of persons with AIDS by category shows that approximately 3 percent of all United States cases do not fit into any identifiable risk group. Doesn't this imply the possibility that AIDS may be transmitted through casual contact?

Once again, there are no documented cases of individuals receiving AIDS through nonsexual contact with saliva, urine, or feces from a person with AIDS or someone in a known risk category. This includes countless health professionals who have been exposed to bodily secretions of AIDS patients. It is noteworthy that the subgroup of persons without known risk factors has been shown to contain many individuals with reported contact with prostitutes, a history of greater than 100 sexual partners, or birth in a country such as Haiti or Central Africa where heterosexual sex is thought to play a major role in AIDS transmission. The body of evidence still points to blood and semen as the major routes of AIDS transmission.

88. Can insects such as mosquitoes transmit AIDS from one person to another?

While this may appear a theoretical possibility, evidence is lacking to support this notion. If the AIDS virus could be transferred from one person to another by insect bite, it seems reasonable to expect a least some cases of AIDS or infection to occur in nonsexual household contacts of persons with AIDS. No such cases have been reported. In addition, the absence of cases in preadolescent children (excluding those in known risk groups) where that age group is prone to direct exposure to many insects also argues against insect transmission of the virus.

It is possible to isolate the AIDS virus from bedbugs one hour after they have been fed blood purposefully contaminated with the AIDS virus. Given the low levels of virus found in human blood and the small volumes that are consumed by insects while biting, the transmission of AIDS virus through this means seems unlikely and is consistent with the lack of reports relating infection to contact wih insects. The hepatitis B virus, which can also be isolated from infected insects and is more easily transmitted than the AIDS virus, has also been shown not to be spread by insects.

89. Doesn't the unusual outbreak of AIDS reported in Palm Beach County, Florida, in 1986 suggest possible transmission by mosquitoes?

From July 1982 to September 1986, 79 cases of AIDS were reported to the CDC from western Palm Beach County, Florida, particularly in residents of the town of Belle Glade. Based on the population census, this incidence was approximately 30 times that expected for a comparable population in the United States.

Because of this unusually high incidence in an area associated with swamps, national television and magazines gave this fact extensive coverage and suggested that mosquito transmission was a possible, albeit unproven, means of AIDS virus transmission.

Investigators from the CDC examined the data from western Palm Beach County and uncovered the following:

- Of the three children with AIDS, all were born to mothers infected with the AIDS virus.
- Of the remaining 76 adults with AIDS, 63 were members of groups known to be at risk for AIDS infection (such as intravenous drug abusers or those having sexual contact with an infected person) or born in countries where heterosexual transmission plays a major role in infection.
- Of the remaining 13 persons without known risk factors, ten died before epidemiological investigation of their risks were completed.
- To indirectly evaluate the exposure to mosquitoes of AIDS virus infected versus uninfected persons, blood was tested for antibodies to five viruses known to be carried by mosquitoes. There was no significant difference in prevalence of antibodies to these viruses between AIDS virus infected and uninfected persons.

Thus, the high incidence of AIDS in western Palm Beach County, Florida, resulted primarily from known risk factors such as use of contaminated needles for injecting illicit drugs intravenously and sexual contact with those in risk groups. Furthermore, those persons infected with the AIDS virus had no greater likelihood than those without AIDS virus infection to be exposed to mosquitoes. The unusually high incidence of AIDS was not related to mosquito transmission.

90. *What is the Haitian link to AIDS?*

Haitians and travelers to Haiti from both Europe and the United States form a small but larger than expected proportion of all AIDS cases. Scientists noted that the first cases of AIDS in Haiti occurred in 1978 and 1979. The epidemiology and presentation of the illness in Haiti resembled that of drug abusers in the United States. Although the high number of Haitians with AIDS initially seemed to hold possible leads to the origin of AIDS, further research suggested that the virus was probably introduced by vacationing Americans or Haitians who had traveled in Central Africa. Haiti has been a desirable vacationing spot for many homosexual men and has a low incidence of antibody positive results in the general population. The clustering of antibody positive individuals around the Carrefour district of Port-au-Prince, which is recognized as the major locale for male and female prostitution in Haiti, suggests that the unusual numbers of Haitians with AIDS may be related to known risk factors that apply to only a limited number of Haitians.

CHAPTER FIVE

Exposure to the AIDS Virus: The Meaning of Antibody Positivity

91. How about receiving blood during surgery or other procedures? How can people protect themselves against AIDS if there have been documented transfusion-associated cases in the past?

On March 2, 1985, the U.S. Food and Drug Administration licensed the first screening test for AIDS virus antibodies. Within one month, virtually all blood bank centers in the United States were using this screening technique. Initial results suggested that 0.25 percent (1 in 400) of the first 1,100,000 units of donated blood gathered in 131 blood centers in the United States between April and June, 1985, showed repeated antibody positivity. This test result is considered evidence of exposure to the AIDS virus. Following a large educational campaign to discourage high risk individuals from donating blood, studies of recent donors show an antibody positivity rate of donated blood approaching 0.01 percent (1 in 10,000). Nevertheless, screening of donated blood for AIDS virus antibody is routine and all units of blood that do show infection with the AIDS virus are discarded.

92. If blood is screened for AIDS antibody, and an individual donates blood, would he be told if he were antibody positive?

The U.S. Public Health Service has recommended that (1) all blood donation facilities notify donors if a repeat antibody test is positive following an initially positive result, that (2) this information should be given in a manner to insure confidentiality of the results and the donor's identity, and that (3) the donor should be referred to a physician for counseling and evaluation given that a positive antibody test result is a preliminary finding and may not represent true infection. A more complete evaluation is warranted for definition of an individual's clinical state.

93. What type of inquiry might the physician be interested in if a person is antibody positive?

The U.S. Public Health Service has suggested repeated testing as the initial step. The physician should investigate the existence of risk factors for AIDS and the presence of medical symptoms that are consistent with AIDS. Tests of lymphocyte function as well as testing for AIDS antibody in the individual's sexual contacts have been recommended as additional sources of information, if clinically warranted.

94. Are there other facilities besides blood donation sites that provide AIDS antibody testing?

A problem identified at blood donation sites was their use by individuals in groups at high risk for AIDS in an effort to learn their antibody status. This ran the possible danger of introducing contaminated blood which slipped through the screening process into the total blood pool. To address this problem, the CDC awarded $9.7 million to 55 areas to set up sites separate from blood donation facilities where confidential antibody testing would be provided at no cost. By December 31, 1985, 874 sites had been established nationwide and over 79,000 persons had been tested. A total of 17.3 percent of the individuals tested at these sites had repeatedly antibody positive test results.

95. Is the AIDS antibody test used to screen blood donors for exposure to the AIDS virus the same that is used in a physician's office to assess for evidence of exposure to the AIDS virus?

Yes. This test can be performed on human blood regardless of whether that blood comes from individuals donating to blood banks or presenting their blood for testing alone; it is not a screening test for AIDS but rather a screening test for infection or exposure to the AIDS virus. However, the fact that the AIDS virus has been isolated from more than 50 percent of healthy antibody positive persons emphasizes the general relationship between antibody positivity and the presence of virus, and the potential for these individuals to infect others.

96. How accurate is the AIDS antibody test for determining exposure to AIDS virus?

As in other laboratory tests designed to detect exposure to infectious agents, inaccurate results can occur due to lab error or to non-specific cross-reactions in the individual being tested. It has been recommended that physicians repeat the antibody test on all individuals who initially have positive test results before reporting such results to the individual. Nevertheless, the finding of high rates of antibody positivity in those groups expected to be at risk for AIDS suggests a direct relationship between antibody positivity and exposure to the AIDS virus.

97. Is there more than one test that measures exposure to the AIDS virus?

There are a variety of tests that have been developed to indicate exposure to AIDS virus. The most commonly used test is called the ELISA (enzyme linked immunosorbent assay). This test uses a color change to indicate presence of the antibody when exposed to certain chemicals. Another test, the Western blot test, can identify antibodies to viral proteins of specific weight. Preliminary data suggest that the ELISA, compared with the Western blot test, is more accurate in correctly identifying those who truly have had AIDS virus exposure (truly antibody positive) and less able to correctly identify those individuals who truly have not had AIDS virus exposure (truly antibody negative). Put another way, if one has had AIDS virus exposure, the ELISA test will more accurately detect this but will also falsely detect exposure in a few other people. If one truly has not had AIDS virus exposure, the Western blot test will more accurately identify this but may also include as negative results a few persons who really have been infected.

98. So, if the Western blot test is less able to accurately identify someone who truly has had AIDS virus exposure, why would someone give that test instead of ELISA?

If an ELISA has positive results, a confirmatory test might be the Western blot test. Because the Western blot test is less sensitive than the ELISA in detecting persons with truly antibody positive results, a positive result supports the conclusion of antibody positivity. A negative Western blot test result following an initially positive ELISA result suggests that the ELISA may have inaccurately identified the person as antibody positive. This inaccuracy can result from antibodies that cross-react in the ELISA test and other sources of error that give weakly positive results that may falsely indicate exposure to the AIDS virus. At the present time, the Western blot test is primarily a research tool and remains too cumbersome and time-consuming to be employed widely as a mass screening technique.

99. Summarize the possibilities a positive ELISA antibody test result can mean for an otherwise healthy appearing person.

- A positive test result may arise either from a technical laboratory error or a reaction to another, similar substance besides the AIDS antibody, falsely suggesting the presence of antibodies to the AIDS virus. It is because of this possibility that repeat ELISA testing and Western blot testing are warranted as confirmatory tests in most individuals.

- A positive test result may indicate that the person has had prior exposure to the AIDS virus but no longer harbors the virus. The person developed antibodies to the virus as the result of the exposure. This situation probably occurs only rarely.

- A positive test result may also indicate that the person has had exposure to the AIDS virus and still harbors the virus. This is the usual interpretation of antibody positivity. It is not known which persons in this group will progress to AIDS or AIDS-related illnesses.

100. Are there limitations to a mass screening program?

Aside from the practical difficulties of the cost and the logistics of screening large numbers of people, the population being screened also affects the accuracy of the test results. A positive antibody test result in a high risk group is more likely to be accurate than a positive antibody result in a low risk group. For example, assume two different populations in which the incidence of AIDS is 1 in 500 in the first and 1 in 50,000 in the second. If the test inaccurately finds 1 in 5,000 of all normal people antibody positive, then in the first population a positive antibody test result would be correct approximately 90 percent of the time, and in the second population, the antibody test would be correct only about 10 percent of the time. Thus, the characteristics of the population being screened must be considered before mass screening results can be properly interpreted.

101. What is the interval between becoming infected with the AIDS virus and first testing antibody positive?

Reports of persons still with antibody negative results years after a known critical exposure (exposure to another infected person through any established means of AIDS virus transmission) strengthens the belief that not everyone with an exposure becomes infected. Among those who do become infected with the AIDS virus, limited case reports suggest that the period of time between acquiring the virus through exposure to an infected person and demonstrating antibody positivity is from one to six months.

102. If an individual is antibody negative, does that mean there is no chance of having the virus?

No. Depending upon the ELISA test used, up to 20 percent of persons with AIDS have shown no evidence of antibody positivity at some time in the course of their illness. There are also a number of reports of individuals with antibody negative results who carry the virus in semen and blood. In fact, a recent study of sex partners of persons with AIDS and ARC showed that four individuals without clinical evidence of disease had antibody negative results but harbored the virus in their lymphocytes.

103. Previously, it was mentioned that 20 percent of persons with AIDS have antibody negative results. Isn't AIDS a condition that, by definition, implies exposure to the virus?

AIDS cannot develop without exposure to the virus. Seronegativity in persons with AIDS probably reflects the inability of the test to detect the antibody rather than the absence of the antibody itself. Also, some studies have shown that in the late terminal stages of AIDS, some persons lose the antibody that was present earlier in their disease.

By late 1985, there were four commercially available ELISAs licensed by the U.S. Food and Drug Administration. They are made by Genetic Systems Corporation, Abbott Laboratories, Organon Teknika, and Electro-Nucleonics. A Red Cross study examined units of blood found to be repeatedly antibody positive by an ELISA test from any of the latter three companies. Further analysis showed that some of these units were inconsistently antibody positive depending on the ELISA test used. The Western blot test more commonly had positive results in detecting the antibody when blood tested antibody positive by more than one ELISA test. This suggests that there is variability in the accuracy of the tests, implying that the test for the presence or absence of the AIDS antibody does not perfectly reflect exposure to the virus.

104. Can an individual be assured that a negative antibody test result means that he or she is not capable of transmitting the virus?

As mentioned before, a small proportion of persons with AIDS have antibody negative results, and there are additional reports of individuals without AIDS who have antibody negative findings but carry and shed the virus from their blood and semen. While these latter reports of antibody negativity in persons known to harbor the virus probably reflect the imperfect ability for antibody testing to detect prior AIDS virus exposure, they support the existence of an antibody-negative carrier state in some seemingly healthy appearing persons.

Recently, 215 sexually active homosexual men without evidence of AIDS were assessed for the presence of antibody positivity. Most of these men had a history of either having had sex with a person with AIDS or over 100 total sexual partners. Of 33 who had antibody negative findings, two had the AIDS virus recovered from their lymphocytes. In June 1986, the CDC documented a case of transfusion-associated transmission of the AIDS virus from a bisexual man who had antibody negative results at the time of donation but later had strongly antibody positive findings. The finding that several healthy persons in high risk groups for AIDS are antibody negative carriers of the AIDS virus strongly emphasizes the need to avoid basing behavioral recommendations to reduce the risk of acquiring or transmitting AIDS solely on the basis of antibody test results.

105. If the antibody test cannot say for certain that a person has or has not been exposed, what value does it have?

The test has utility in screening blood products that are repeatedly positive and can be discarded from the transfusion pool. The test also has value for individuals who are in high risk groups in which the probability that a positive test result really is true is greater than in a low risk group. An antibody test may influence an individual to alter his or her lifestyle once that person realizes he or she may spread the virus or may not yet have been exposed. Individuals who have difficult-to-define medical symptoms may have clarification of their illness with a positive test result. Additionally, the antibody test is also an important public health tool. By continuing to screen populations, scientists can track the appearance of the virus into places where it was not previously found and thereby stimulate the public health precautions necessary to minimize virus transmission.

The difficult problem in interpreting the AIDS antibody test for individual use is the possibility that an inaccurate positive result might radically alter that person's life and that an inaccurate negative result might lull one into a false sense of security where one misses the opportunity to employ precautions that minimize infection of others. Important public policy decisions will undoubtedly have to be made concerning the recommended use of antibody testing in a manner that balances the information made useful to the individual with that made useful to the population at large. The recent announcement that a new antibody test developed jointly by Genetic Systems Corporation in Seattle and the Pasteur Institute in Paris correctly detected antibodies in 100 percent of tested AIDS patients and incorrectly reported antibody positivity in only 0.2 percent (1 in 150) of nonrisk group donors suggests the pending availability of increasingly accurate tests to determine exposure to the AIDS virus.

106. If a person is antibody positive, should he or she be considered infectious and capable of transmitting the virus even if there are no symptoms of disease?

Yes. Although it is clear that more studies are needed that follow antibody positive individuals over time and that record the incidence of AIDS in these people, it is also clear that a small proportion of antibody positive individuals with no symptoms of disease have transmitted the AIDS virus to their sexual partners.

The most convincing evidence of the infectivity of antibody-positive persons comes from studying blood donors who were implicated as the sources of infection for persons developing AIDS after receiving a transfusion. Twenty-three donors, all healthy, with antibody positive results, and free of AIDS, gave blood samples to researchers from one to five years after their original blood donation. All donors had the AIDS virus isolated and grown from their lymphocytes. Medical experts have recommeded that all individuals with antibody positive findings be considered potentially capable of infecting others.

107. How long can a person remain infected and asymptomatic?

It may be the case that many individuals with antibody positive results will remain asymptomatic their entire lives. The blood of hemophiliacs has been retrospectively tested for presence of AIDS antibody and shows several hemophiliacs remaining asymptomatic during seven years of antibody positivity.

108. What ability, then, does the antibody test have to predict the occurrence of disease?

The antibody test has very limited ability to predict disease. Since most information on people with antibody positive or negative results and their respective outcomes was determined in high risk groups, the significance of having antibody positive findings can only be extrapolated for other groups. It is known that among homosexual men with antibody positive results but without symptoms of AIDS, more than 60 percent remained disease-free when followed over a two to five year period. It may be argued that those who remained asymptomatic, in fact, represent individuals with longer incubation periods between exposure and onset of the disease compared to those already with AIDS. It may also be true that many individuals who have antibody positive results may remain AIDS-free their entire lives.

Much scientific attention has been turned to understanding the events that might precede or cause a person to develop signs of AIDS or one of its related disorders once a person is infected. Theories have been proposed implicating a variety of as yet unidentified co-factors that might hasten the appearance of disease in an infected person. Time and careful data collection will be needed to fully understand the significance of having antibody positivity to the AIDS virus and how other factors influence the risk of developing AIDS.

109. In summary, then, what is the relationship between having antibody positive results and the risk of getting AIDS?

Accurately predicting the risk of developing AIDS from the finding of antibody positivity is difficult. What is known is that in high risk populations, the number of persons with antibody positive results is much greater than the number of persons with AIDS. It is estimated that this ratio is between 50:1 and 100:1 and that at least from 7 to 25 percent of antibody positive individuals will later develop AIDS or related syndromes. This estimate is based on retrospective reviews of individuals with antibody positive results and their development of the disease over a four-year period. However, estimates for longer periods are difficult to make because of the known lengthy incubation period of the disease. While this incubation period is estimated to be an average of three years based on those who had a single exposure to the virus through a blood transfusion and their subsequent development of AIDS, the actual figure may be longer. This is because the disease has not been recognized long enough to incorporate those cases with a longer incubation period which will manifest themselves with increasing time. The recent report of AIDS in a child 5.5 years after a single transfusion suggests that more definitive answers about incubation time and the risk for AIDS of asymptomatic individuals with antibody positive results must await the passage of time. It is also of note that scientists have demonstrated the ability of the AIDS virus to infect T-helper lymphocytes in the absence of cell death, suggesting an in vitro model for the long latency between virus exposure and disease onset in many affected individuals.

110. Are there any factors present in some people that influence or predict the course of infection with HIV?

Researchers have identified a group of people with repeated unprotected exposure to HIV-infected individuals that does not develop evidence of infection with HIV. A genetic analysis indicated that members of this group could frequently be distinguished from infected individuals by the presence in their blood of a specific type of serum protein called group component. Three different forms of group component have been identified in humans, but only those individuals that have the form called Gc2 have a reduced chance of becoming infected with HIV after exposure to the virus. The Gc2 protein is not absolutely protective against infection with HIV, and its exact role in slowing or preventing the progression of disease to AIDS once a person is infected is undetermined at this point. How Gc2 hinders HIV infection is not yet clear, but it may be that it interferes with binding of the virus to the surface of susceptible cells.

Approximately 10 percent of the population has genes for only Gc2, and another 39 percent has combinations of genes for Gc2 and the different forms of Gc1. The finding of a genetically determined susceptibility to infection with HIV is an important lead in understanding the relative risks for infection in exposed individuals, but it is premature at this time to ascribe the lower rates of HIV infection in individuals with the Gc2 protein solely to the presence of the protein. It may well be that the protein is only a marker for some other factor that influences infection. Given that Gc-typing is a research tool done in a limited number of laboratories in the world, determination of an individual's Gc type is not yet a routine practice. The exact relationship of the presence of Gc2 to the risk of HIV infection and the development of AIDS remains to be defined.

Another study has found that other factors appear to be predictive of an increased likelihood of developing AIDS in individuals already infected with HIV.

In a study of 1,835 homosexual men who had antibody positive findings, AIDS developed in 59 during a follow-up period of approximately 15 months. After many variables were analyzed, attempts were made to identify factors initially present in both groups that could later distinguish the 59 men from the remaining 1,776 who did not develop AIDS.

The factors that were independently associated with an infected person's risk of developing AIDS were:

- a decreased number of T-helper lymphocytes
- an increased number of T-suppressor lymphocytes
- a low level of antibody to the AIDS virus
- a high level of antibody against cytomegalovirus
- a history of sex with someone in whom AIDS developed

While these factors correlated with an infected person's increased risk of developing AIDS, they may represent factors that are markers rather than determinants of disease progression. In addition, the study of homosexual men in this report makes the relevance of these findings to other groups of persons infected with the AIDS virus uncertain.

111. What are some precautions recommended for a person with antibody positive results to decrease the risk of virus transmission to others?

Avoiding the sharing of needles among intravenous drug users and reducing one's number of sexual partners will lessen the likelihood of virus transmission to others. It is also recommended that infected persons not share razors, toothbrushes, or any objects potentially contaminated with their blood. In addition, it is prudent to inform physicians, dentists, other health professionals and intimate physical contacts so that appropriate precautions can be taken to minimize accidental transmission of the AIDS virus. Previous sex partners and persons with whom needles have been shared should be encouraged to seek antibody testing. Avoiding the donation of organs, sperm, or other tissues is also recommended.

112. If an individual is planning a family and is antibody positive, is it safe to get pregnant?

The U.S. Public Health Service has recommended that women with AIDS or antibody positivity delay pregnancy to avoid possible transmission of AIDS to the fetus. Women who are unaware of their antibody status but who have been exposed to high risk individuals either through sexual contact or sharing of needles are advised to have a screening test for AIDS antibody before considering pregnancy.

113. Aside from the possibility of transmitting AIDS to the fetus, will antibody positivity pose any added risks to the pregnant woman?

It has been suggested that the normal decrease in immune function that accompanies pregnancy may increase an already infected woman's risk of acquiring AIDS. Pregnancy has long been associated with a decrease in immune function and an increased risk of acquiring certain infections. Before the development of the polio vaccine, for example, pregnant women were not only more susceptible to the disease but had a higher death rate once the illness was contracted. The worldwide spread of the Asian influenza virus in 1957 affected pregnant women with unusual frequency and severity. Studies have shown that the T-lymphocyte helper-to-suppressor ratio is decreased in women during pregnancy and for several months following childbirth.

Fifteen pregnant women with antibody positive results were followed for an average of 2.5 years after the birth of their children. Five of these women developed AIDS, seven developed AIDS-related conditions, and only three remained without symptoms of disease. While this sample size was small and the results may not be applicable to all infected women who are pregnant, they do suggest an increased risk of developing AIDS when pregnancy and infection with the AIDS virus coexist.

114. Has AIDS antibody screening been considered as an optional part of the required rubella-syphilis premarital blood test?

The proposed use of antibody testing in this setting will undoubtedly be a topic for debate among public health workers and legislators.

115. Although it is clear that AIDS is associated with a profound deficiency in immunity, does antibody positivity in a person without AIDS imply any deficiency in immune functioning?

A high proportion of persons without AIDS but infected with the AIDS virus may have immunological abnormalities. A recent study followed healthy homosexual men over a three-year period and assessed clinical history, antibody status, and T-helper/suppressor lymphocyte ratios, considered to be an important indicator of immune function. Complete follow-up data were available for 19 men with antibody positive results and 31 with antibody negative findings. At the end of the three-year period, only four of the 31 (12 percent) men with antibody negative findings had an inverted T-helper/suppressor lymphocyte ratio (less than 1.0), which is considered evidence of impaired immunity. In contrast, 16 of the 19 (92 percent) men with antibody positive results had inverted lymphocyte ratios. Just as important, the longer an individual had antibody positivity, the lower his T-lymphocyte ratio was. Not only the mere presence of the viral infection but also the length of time the person had been infected was associated with immune deficiency.

Another line of evidence that relies on the incidence of tuberculosis indirectly suggests that those infected with the AIDS virus but without evidence of AIDS may have impaired immune systems. Tuberculosis is a disease principally of the lungs and caused by the bacterium Mycobacterium tuberculosis. In most people infected with the tuberculosis bacterium, no symptoms occur because the bacteria are held in check by the immune system. When factors that favor decreased immunity occur, such as old age, certain diseases, or use of immunosuppressive drugs, there is a markedly increased chance of the tuberculosis bacteria becoming active, disseminating, and producing clinical manifestations of disease. In early 1986, the CDC reported that the significant yearly decline in the incidence of tuberculosis that had been occurring since the early 1970s had not taken place during 1985.

The suspicion that infection with the AIDS virus in those without clinical manifestations of AIDS may have been responsible for this trend derived from the following observations.

- Some of the areas that showed an increase in tuberculosis deaths during 1985 (New York, California, Florida, Texas) were also areas with the largest number of AIDS cases and persons with antibody positive findings.
- Since other medical conditions that result in immune deficiency are associated with reactivation of preexisting Mycobacterium tuberculosis infection, there is a theoretical reason to suspect that compromised immunity from infection with the AIDS virus may favor such a reactivation.

- In New York City, there has been an increased number of persons with intravenous drug abuse, a risk factor for acquiring AIDS virus infection, who have been diagnosed with tuberculosis.
- In Florida, a large percentage of persons with AIDS either had tuberculosis at the time AIDS was diagnosed or within an 18-month period preceding the diagnosis.

Additional data are currently being collected in an effort to evaluate to what degree, if any, lymphocyte levels or helper/suppressor ratios in asymptomatic infected persons predict the future development of AIDS.

116. Can life insurance companies require an individual to obtain AIDS antibody testing as a condition for granting insurance?

As of early 1987, California, Connecticut, Florida, Maine, New Jersey, Wisconsin, and Washington, DC have laws prohibiting the use of AIDS antibody testing for this purpose. However, insurance companies may request this testing in other areas where they sell policies, and eight major companies sought approval in late 1986 to require testing in selected applicants. Those who test antibody positive would be denied life insurance by these companies. Other companies are considering proposals to grant insurance to persons with antibody positive findings but at increased cost.

While a number of insurance companies have requested permission to ask questions about AIDS risk and require antibody testing for selected applicants, these requests will be handled on a state-to-state basis. At the present time, the Michigan Insurance Bureau has denied permission to insurance companies to make such an inquiry. In Maryland, on the other hand, a state task force has recommended that insurance carriers be allowed to request antibody testing in certain applicants and to ask questions concerning AIDS on applications.

117 What is the prevalence of the AIDS antibody among different groups?

The following rates of antibody positivity represent data from a number of different studies based on information collected in 1985 and 1986. The ranges within each group reflect differences in these studies. Because the size of some groups studied was relatively small, these figures are expected to be modified as larger study samples become available for testing. Unless otherwise noted, the populations sampled are from the United States.

Groups	Prevalence of Antibody Positive (Percent)
Persons with AIDS	68–100
Persons with AIDS-related illnesses such as ARC or GLS	84–100
Randomly tested homosexual men	17–67
Intravenous drug abusers	
NY City	59–87
New Jersey < 5 miles from NYC	56
New Jersey, 5–10 miles from NYC	43
Edinburgh, Scotland	51
New Haven, CT	10
San Francisco	9
New Jersey, > 100 miles from NYC	2
Persons with hemophilia	
Factor VIII concentrate recipients	74
Factor IX concentrate recipients	39
Cryoprecipitate only recipients	17–40
Female prostitutes, United States	5-40
Female prostitues, Kenya	31-66

Female sexual partners of men with antibody positive findings but asymptomatic	10
Haitians	4-8
Blood donors Female	0.001 (or 1 in 10,000)
Male and female, Connecticut	0.0084 (1 in 10,000)

118. The military is currently testing all recruits for the AIDS antibody. How will this be done and what will be done with the results?

The military is in the process of testing recruits and all 2.1 million military personnel for the AIDS antibody. Their protocol involves initial testing with the ELISA antibody test, which will be repeated if it has positive findings. If the repeat test is also positive, a Western blot antibody test will be given. Recruits with antibody positive results by both tests will be denied entrance to the military. Of the 789,578 recruits tested between October 1985 and January 1987, 1,186 or 0.15 percent (15 per 10,000) had antibody positive findings.

Data on antibody positivity of those already in the military is unavailable. However, it is known that those individuals in the military who test antibody positive and are without evidence of disease will be kept in the service but restricted in their duties and geographic assignments. Other military personnel who have evidence of AIDS or AIDS-related illness will be given available treatment and honorable medical discharges. Because a recent study suggested that 15 of 41 military men with AIDS or ARC were most likely exposed to the virus through sexual contact with high risk partners of the opposite sex and/or prostitutes, educational programs have recently begun to receive high priority by the military.

119. Who should be tested for AIDS antibody positivity?

In an effort to reduce the risk of AIDS transmission, the CDC has strongly recommended voluntary testing for individuals in the following risk groups: homosexual and bisexual men, current or past intravenous drug abusers, persons with signs or symptoms compatible with AIDS or AIDS-related complex, people born in Haiti, Central Africa, and other countries where heterosexual sex is thought to play a major role in the transmission of AIDS, male or female prostitutes and their sexual partners, hemophiliacs who have received blood clotting factors, sexual partners of infected people or of people in the preceding risk groups, and newborn infants of high risk or infected mothers. In addition, those individuals donating organs, tissues, or sperm, not only blood itself, should be tested for exposure to AIDS virus in an effort to prevent transmission; regardless of the results, however, persons in high risk groups should avoid donation of blood, tissues, or sperm.

120. AIDS seems to be a disease that could potentially affect anyone. What can be done to decrease the risk of contracting AIDS?

Blood bank screening tests exist to protect individuals needing a transfusion. Additionally, a wide range of recommendations have been previously mentioned for hemophiliacs in an effort to reduce the incidence of transmission of AIDS through clotting factors. Sexual contact with those at risk for AIDS and the sharing of dirty needles for drug use remain the two principal methods of acquiring AIDS. In March 1983, the U.S. Public Health Service recommended that members of high risk groups reduce their number of sexual partners in an effort to minimize the risk to others of acquiring AIDS. In addition, the use of condoms appears to be another, although as yet unproven, means to reduce the risk of transmitting or acquiring AIDS. The CDC has emphasized that, without an available vaccine or effective therapy, risk reduction is the key to decreasing the spread of AIDS.

It appears that individuals are taking increased precautions, as other sexually transmitted diseases among homosexuals and heterosexuals have been greatly reduced in the last several years. For example, the incidence of gonorrhea in homosexually active men in the Seattle-King County area decreased by 57 percent from 1982 to 1984, compared with a 20 percent

decrease among heterosexual men and women. In San Francisco, data from the City Health Department showed a 73
percent decrease in rectal gonorrhea in men from 1980 to
1984. Since sexual contact remains the primary route of transmission, reducing the number of sexual partners and wearing
condoms during sexual activity can be expected to decrease
one's probability of acquiring the AIDS virus.

121. If, in fact, individuals are becoming less promiscuous and the incidence of sexually transmitted diseases has been decreasing, why has the prevalence of the AIDS antibody been increasing?

Consider the example of gonorrhea. This sexually transmissible disease has had a declining incidence in the last few years,
largely as the result of individual changes in sexual behavior
presumably resulting from fear of contracting AIDS. Because
cases of gonorrhea become clinically apparent more quickly
and are more easily recognized than AIDS virus infection or
many of the other AIDS-related conditions, identification and
treatment of the affected person with gonorrhea is easier.
AIDS, on the other hand, has a longer incubation period and
is not treatable, and there are many asymptomatic virus carriers. Therefore, identification and treatment of all individuals
who are potential sources for transmitting the disease is very
difficult.

For example, in Seattle, approximately one-third of homosexual and bisexual men attending the Sexually Transmitted
Diseases Clinic at Harborview Hospital in 1984 were shown
to be antibody positive for the AIDS virus. Dramatically
changing one's sexual behavior from 40 contacts per year to 4
would be expected to significantly reduce a more identifiable
disease such as gonorrhea. However, given that one-third of
contacts have had exposure to the AIDS virus, the probability
of randomly contacting at least one of these antibody positive
individuals in a sexual encounter would only decrease from
near 100 percent with 40 "chances" or sexual contacts to 81
percent with 4 contacts. Finally, unlike many sexually transmitted diseases, AIDS can be spread via routes other than
sexual ones, making changes in sexual behavior only one pre-
ventive measure against contracting the disease. Other high

risk activities can still transmit the virus and will continue to account for many persons developing antibody positivity.

122. What other evidence exists that changes in sexual behavior have occurred in the male homosexual population?

In an August 1984 telephone survey of randomly selected individuals in San Francisco, self-identified homosexual men and bisexual men were asked questions concerning their sexual behavior. Sixty-nine percent stated that they were monogamous or celibate, and did not engage in anal intercourse without a condom or participate in oral intercourse outside of a primary relationship. Eight months later, these same individuals were recontacted and 81 percent reported the above behaviors. However, at that time it was noteworthy that 7 percent of all respondents in the survey reported oral sex with exchange of semen and 12 percent reported anal intercourse without a condom, both with secondary partners in the previous month. Thirty-six percent of all respondents continued to count more than one sex partner in the previous 30 days.

123. Are the use of condoms, diaphragms, or spermicides protective against contracting AIDS virus infection?

There is good evidence that condoms, diaphragms, and spermicides may play protective roles against AIDS virus transmission. When five different types of condoms were tested in the laboratory, the AIDS virus did not pass through the condom membranes. In addition, several studies have shown that an ingredient in many spermicides inactivates the AIDS virus. Although the effect of diaphragm use on AIDS virus transmission has not been assessed, epidemiological studies have shown a reduced incidence of other sexually transmissible diseases in women who use this device. It is assumed that the protective effect of diaphragms is, as in condoms, due to their roles as mechanical barriers against the offending microorganism. Concurrent use of a spermicide with a diaphragm, therefore, may be expected to provide added protection against AIDS virus transmission.

The laboratory setting where condom and spermicide testing occurs cannot simulate real-life use of these devices and take into account the potential hazards of mechanical failure and other variables. For example, sperm has also been shown to be incapable of penetrating the membranes of condoms in test tube settings; yet, epidemiological studies have shown that as many as 10 percent of women whose partners use condoms still become pregnant. Although the use of condoms, diaphragms, and spermicides seems like a logical measure to take to decrease one's risk of acquiring or transmitting the AIDS virus, it should not be regarded as complete protection at the present time.

124. If both sex partners are infected with the AIDS virus but do not have AIDS, will continued sexual contact with each other increase the risk of acquiring AIDS?

It is unknown whether reinfection with the AIDS virus causes already infected persons to increase their risk of acquiring AIDS. Since the risk is not known, it has been suggested that infected couples take precautions by using condoms and spermicides during sexual intercourse.

CHAPTER SIX

Protecting the Individual and Health Care Worker

125. What is known about the risk to health care workers of acquiring AIDS or infection in the workplace?

No health care worker has contracted AIDS from the casual contact or other occupational exposures associated with caring for a patient. Regarding the risk of acquiring infection, five separate studies examined over 1,498 health care workers. Included in this group were 666 individuals who had direct needle-stick or mucous membrane exposure to the blood or bodily fluid of patients with either AIDS or antibody positivity. Only 26 or 1.7 percent of the entire group of health care workers were antibody positive and all but 3 of these 26 belonged to risk groups for AIDS. Of the 3 workers not in any defined risk group, no specific occupational exposures outside of accidental self-inoculation with a dirty needle could be documented.

A recent study prospectively examined those health care workers who accidentally stuck themselves with a needle used in the care of an AIDS patient. It is noteworthy that after an eight month follow-up period, none of the 105 individuals have had antibody positive findings. Although it is early in the follow-up period, these preliminary data suggest that antibody conversion is infrequent in the population of general health care workers, even when those with known direct exposures are included.

126. What is known about the risk to household members of acquiring AIDS or infection from the care of persons with AIDS at home?

As with health care workers, there have been no reported cases of AIDS or infection related to casual contact in household members intimately involved in the care of family members with AIDS. However, the CDC has recently reported the apparent transmission of the AIDS virus from a child to his mother who was providing health care for him at home.

The child, a two-year-old boy, was born with a congenital disorder that required multiple surgeries and resulted in many episodes of bleeding and transfusions during his 17 months in the hospital. During his hospitalization, he was noted to have antibody positive findings. Samples from 26 of the donors whose blood had been transfused to him were retrospectively tested and one was found to be strongly antibody positive. Following the child's release home, his mother became intimately involved in his care, which resulted in multiple contacts with his blood and feces. Because the child had indwelling intravenous tubing allowing direct access to his bloodstream, the mother had frequent exposure to blood during his care. Although the mother could not recall any needlesticks, her hands were contaminated with blood, saliva, and bloody feces on multiple occasions. She admitted to not regularly washing her hands after contacting the child and she did not wear gloves while working with the child or while handling his contaminated urine and feces. She was documented to have antibody negative results before converting to antibody positivity. In addition, she appeared to have no risk factors beyond the care of her child, and her husband had antibody negative findings with normal T-helper-to-suppressor lymphocyte ratios. Thus, this woman most likely acquired her AIDS virus infection from her son while providing intensive nursing care involving contact with blood.

Although such exposure cannot be considered casual or even typical of the type of exposure household members have to family members with AIDS, it strongly emphasizes the importance to health care workers and others of following CDC guidelines, such as wearing gloves in hospital, institutional, or home settings where blood or bodily secretions of persons with AIDS are routinely handled.

A related series of cases was reported to the CDC in mid-1987 when three health care workers developed antibodies to the AIDS virus following single exposures of their skin to large amounts of HIV-infected blood. In all cases, the integrity of the health care workers' skin was noted to be compromised by dermatitis, acne, or chapping, and in all instances standard CDC guidelines recommending the use of gloves with exposure to blood were not followed. There is no evidence at present to suggest that the proper use of gloves and the protection of damaged skin will fail to protect against infection with HIV.

127. In what other ways can individuals protect themselves in the hospital or home setting?

Health care workers and persons caring for those with AIDS at home should continue to employ the same precautions used to avoid contracting other viral diseases transmissible through blood and semen, such as hepatitis B. These include wearing gloves when handling bodily fluids or touching mucous membranes or nonintact skin of all patients, using care when performing any blood-related procedure to prevent injuries to hands caused by needles or other sharp instruments, covering any area of oneself where skin has been broken, careful hand washing, and following established hospital and CDC guidelines for disposal of dirty needles, blood products, and other contaminants from any patient.

128. Is there anything that can be done if someone is accidentally stuck with a needle that has been used on a person with AIDS?

There is currently no specific treatment against the virus in any phase of its infectious cycle.

129. Can AIDS be acquired through exposure to the tears of a person with AIDS?

There has been no case to date of AIDS caused by exposure to tears. However, workers at the National Institutes of Health have isolated the virus from the tears of a woman with AIDS who had no eye abnormalities. In addition, the AIDS virus has been recovered from soft contact lenses worn by three of six patients studied. The CDC has therefore developed recommendations to avoid the passage of virus through tears. They include (1) careful handwashing by health care workers after examining patients; gloves are advisable when there is a break in the examiner's skin, (2) instruments that contact the eye such as those used to test for glaucoma should be treated with hydrogen peroxide or a chlorinated solution, (3) contact lenses should be disinfected between trial fittings by either hydrogen peroxide or heat treatments.

130. If accidently stuck with a needle from a patient, what legal right does a person have either to force the patient to undergo antibody testing or to obtain the results of prior testing?

The jurisdiction to enact laws addressing this question rests with each state. In California and Wisconsin, it is illegal to force another individual to undergo antibody testing and to reveal information about an individual's antibody status to anybody other than a health care worker providing direct medical care. The issue of whether a health care worker has the right in special circumstances to obtain information on the antibody status of a particular patient is presently being addressed in the courts through litigation.

131. Is it possible to obtain AIDS from cardiopulmonary resuscitation mannequins? How about actual mouth-to-mouth resuscitation?

The Scientific Advisory Panel on Emergency Medicine, Internal Medicine, and Preventative Medicine and Public Health has verified the absence of AIDS cases from the use of cardiopulmonary resuscitation mannequins. No known case of transmission of AIDS or AIDS virus through saliva or mouth-to-mouth resuscitation has been documented. Recently, data concerning two nurses who performed mouth-to-mouth resuscitation on an AIDS patient became available. At an eight-month follow-up period, the nurses continued to have antibody negative results with normal T-helper-to-suppressor ratios.

Because the AIDS virus has been found in saliva, the theoretical possibility exists that saliva may be a route of virus transmissibility during intimate salivary exchange. Many paramedics have been equipped with special resuscitation masks to avoid actual contact and minimize this possibility. It has also been recommended that a disposable ventilating bag be kept at the bedside of each patient with AIDS or an AIDS-related illness to avoid mucous-membrane exposure in the event of a cardiopulmonary arrest.

132. If saliva is a theoretically possible mode of transmitting the AIDS virus, can AIDS be contracted by sharing eating and drinking utensils?

Unlike the intimate salivary exchange across mucous membranes that can occur in deep kissing, the risk of acquiring AIDS from eating and drinking from common utensils appears to be near zero and no such cases have occurred. Nevertheless, fear of acquiring AIDS through this means has been addressed by some. For example, clergy at the National Cathedral in Washington, DC, have changed their procedure for Holy Communion in response to growing concerns about AIDS and an associate decline in the number of parishioners taking Communion. Rather than drinking wine from a common chalice, parishioners now have the option of accepting a wafer dipped in wine held in a container from which no one drinks; approximately 50 percent of the communicants now use this alternative.

133. What risks do infected food-service workers play in transmitting the AIDS virus?

All evidence suggests that the AIDS virus has not been spread by persons through the preparation and serving of food. The risk of food exposed to blood through cuts can be minimized by the wearing of gloves by the food handler. Although AIDS virus has been isolated in saliva, nonsexual transmission of the virus through saliva has not been noted and handling of food by an infected worker who adheres to routine good hygiene is expected to present no risk to the customer.

134. Is it true that AIDS has been acquired by women through artificial insemination?

Cases of four Australian women artificially inseminated with semen from a carrier of the AIDS virus have been reported. These women had no known risk factors for AIDS. As of 1986, three years after insemination, one of the four had developed GLS while the others have remained disease-free. The finding that an AIDS-related disease can be acquired through artificial insemination adds further support to the role of semen in the transmission of AIDS virus. It has also resulted in sperm banks reevaluating storage techniques and donor requirements in an effort to minimize AIDS virus transmission during artificial insemination.

Approximately 30,000 to 60,000 artificial inseminations are performed yearly in the United States, and 6,000 to 10,000 live births result. At the present time, rapid, accurate testing of sperm for AIDS virus is unavailable. Instead, many sperm banks and fertility clinics utilize the following protocol to minimize AIDS virus transmission during artificial insemination: (1) sperm donors are tested for antibody positivity at the time of donation, (2) because of the lag time between infection with the AIDS virus and testing antibody positive, sperm donors are retested two to four months later, (3) the semen is frozen at the time of initial donation and not used until the second donor test is shown to be negative.

Although the chance of a successful pregnancy is lowered by about 10 to 15 percent with the use of frozen rather than fresh semen, the advantages to the mother and her fetus of retesting the sperm donor for AIDS antibody positivity before sperm is used appear to be great.

135. What are adequate disinfecting procedures for linen, clothes, medical instruments, etc., used by a person with AIDS or with antibody positivity?

The following procedures will inactivate the AIDS virus:

Medical instruments contaminated with blood or body fluids: chemical germicides such as 25% ethanol (for five minutes); or 1% gluteraldehyde; or autoclaving when materials permit.

Medical instruments that contact the eye: five-to-ten minute exposure to 3% hydrogen peroxide, or a 1:10 part solution of household bleach, or 70% ethanol, or 70% isopropanol. The instruments should be rinsed thoroughly in tap water before reuse.

Contact lenses: soft: hydrogen peroxide, or heat disinfecting at 172 degrees F for ten minutes; *rigid gas permeable:* hydrogen peroxide; *hard:* hydrogen peroxide.

Linen, clothes, glassware, and utensils: laundry and dishwashing cycles commonly used in hospital settings.

Environmental surfaces exposed to blood: household bleach diluted 1:10 in water (0.5% concentration of sodium hypochlorite) or 70% alcohol.

136. Many medical patients have conditions such as malnutrition and are treated with drugs that can depress immunity. Do these factors increase their susceptibility to AIDS?

AIDS is an acquired, transmissible disease. The crucial factor in a person contracting AIDS is an exposure to the AIDS virus. It may be true that once infected, nutritional, behavioral, and genetic factors that affect immunity and are unique to the individual may increase the probability of an infected person acquiring AIDS. This is speculative and derives from examples of many infectious diseases in which the course is influenced by such predisposing factors. Due to this concern, it has been recommended that physicians exercise caution in using immunosuppressive drugs such as steroids in patients with risk factors for AIDS. It is also clear that previously healthy young persons without any coexisting factors that depress immunity have contracted the AIDS virus, and developed its progressive, terminal complications.

137. Should a pregnant woman be involved in the care of a person with AIDS?

A pregnant woman having nonsexual, casual contact with a person with AIDS runs no risk of her fetus acquiring AIDS, as

she herself is not at risk for AIDS infection through this exposure. However, those with AIDS are susceptible to infection
from a variety of microorganisms such as cytomegalovirus.
Because a few of these microorganisms can be transmitted
through casual contact, can infect the healthy mother, and are
capable of producing severe disease in fetuses while the
mother remains asymptomatic, it is recommended that pregnant women not be directly involved in the care of persons
with AIDS.

138. Are transplant recipients at risk for AIDS?

There have been five case reports relating the probable transmission of the AIDS virus to patients through transplanted
kidneys. Each kidney recipient had not developed AIDS at the
time of the case report but had strongly positive AIDS antibody findings. Additionally, it was known that each patient
had antibody negative results prior to transplantation and had
no known risk factors for exposure to the virus. Four of the
five donors from whom the transplanted kidney was obtained
were intravenous drug abusers. Individuals who are antibody
positive or in high risk groups should refrain from donation of
any organ for transplantation.

139. Are there other medical practices that could potentially
pass the virus from one person to another?

Much study has centered on the risk of blood transfusions and
blood products in passage of the virus from an infected donor
to an uninfected recipient. A variety of other practices that
may employ the use of unclean needles or other unsterile instruments to puncture the skin are potential sources of virus
spread. Examples of such practices include ear piercing, ta-
tooing, male or female circumcision, blood-brotherhood cere-
monies, and, as in the case of intravenous drug abusers,
injections with unsterile needles.

Although case reports are lacking, the rapid increase in the
prevalence of persons in the general population with antibody
positive findings suggests that with the passage of time cases
as the result of the aforementioned routes of inoculation will

appear. In Africa there are now data that implicate multiple injections with unsterile needles as an increasingly common way to transmit the virus.

140. Summarize where the AIDS virus is found and how it is transmitted.

Body Site	Presence of AIDS Virus	Possible Modes of Transmissibility
Blood	Yes	sharing of contaminated intravenous needles; receiving infected blood transfusions; receiving infected blood products; maternal-fetal placental transfer
Brain tissue	Yes	
Breast milk	Yes	maternal-child transmission
Cerebrospinal fluid	Yes	
Feces	Yes	
Saliva	Yes	? exchange of saliva through intimate kissing*
Skin	No	
Sperm	Yes	artificial insemination; genital to oral, anal, or vaginal routes
Tears	Yes	*
Urine	Yes	*
Vaginal secretions	Yes	genital to oral* or genital to genital

*Unproven as route of virus transmission.

141. The presence of children with AIDS in schools has been a complex and controversial medical-legal-social dilemma. What recommendations has the U.S. Public Health Service made to educators and parents of school-aged children?

After consulting with the Conference of State and Territorial Epidemiologists, the Association of State and Territorial Health Officials, the National Association for Elementary School Principals, the Division of Maternal and Child Health, the National Association of School Nurse Consultants, the National Congress of Parents and Teachers, and the Children's Aid Society, the U.S. Public Health Service has made the following recommendations regarding AIDS among school-aged children. In considering issues that interface law and medicine, special attention was given to issues of civil rights and assessment of transmissibility and risks for all parties. These recommendations were:

- Decisions regarding the type of education and care should be based on the behavior, neurological development, and physical condition of the child and the expected type of interaction with others in that setting. These decisions are best made using a team approach including the child's physician, public health personnel, the child's parent or guardian, and personnel associated with the proposed care or educational setting. In each case, risks and benefits to both the infected child and others in the setting should be weighed.
- For *most* infected school-aged children, the benefits of an unrestricted school setting outweigh the disadvantages. These disadvantages include the risk of the AIDS child acquiring potentially harmful infections from others and the apparent nonexistent risk of transmission of the AIDS virus to other school children. Children with AIDS, therefore, should be allowed to attend school and after-school day care in unrestricted settings.
- For the (1) infected preschool-aged child, (2) some neurologically handicapped children who lack control of their body secretions or who display behavior such as biting, and (3) those children who have uncoverable, oozing lesions, a more restricted environment is advis-

able until more is known about transmission in these settings.

- Care involving exposure to the infected child's body fluids and exrement, such as feeding and diaper changing, should be performed by persons who are aware of the child's infection and the modes of possible transmission. In any setting involving an AIDS-infected person good handwashing after exposure to blood and body fluids and before caring for another child should be observed. Gloves should be worn if open lesions are present on the caretaker's hands. Any open lesions on the infected person should also be covered.

- Because other infections in addition to AIDS can be present in blood or body fluids, all schools and day care facilities, regardless of whether children with AIDS infection are attending, should adopt routine procedures for handling blood or body fluids. Soiled surfaces should be cleaned promptly with disinfectant, such as household bleach (diluted 1 part bleach to 10 parts water). Disposable towels or tissues should be used whenever possible, and mops should be rinsed in the disinfectant. Those who are cleaning should avoid exposure of open skin lesions or mucous membranes such as those in the mouth to blood or body fluids of an infected person.

- The hygienic practices of children with AIDS infection may improve as the child matures. Alternatively, the hygienic practices may deteriorate if the child's condition worsens. Evaluation to assess the need for a restricted environment should be performed regularly.

- Physicians caring for children born to mothers with AIDS or at increased risk of acquiring AIDS infection should consider testing the children for evidence of AIDS virus infection for medical reasons. For example, vaccination of infected children with virus vaccines such as the measles-mumps-rubella vaccine may be hazardous. These children also need to be followed closely for problems with growth and development and given prompt and aggressive therapy for infections and exposure to potentially lethal infections, such as varicella (chicken pox). In the event that an antiviral agent or other therapy for AIDS infection becomes available, these children should be considered for such therapy. Knowledge that the child is infected, regardless of whether he does or does not have symptoms, will allow parents and other caretakers to take precautions when exposed to the blood and body fluids of the child.

· Adoption and foster care agencies should consider adding AIDS antibody screening to the routine medical evaluation of children at increased risk of infection before placement in the foster or adoptive home, since these parents must make decisions regarding the care of the child and must consider the possible social and psychological effects on their families.

· Mandatory screening for AIDS antibody as a condition for school entry is not warranted based on available data.

· Persons involved in the care and education of AIDS-infected children should respect the child's right to privacy, including maintaining confidential records. The number of personnel who are aware of the child's condition should be kept at the minimum needed to assure proper care of the child and to detect situations where the potential for transmission may increase (such as a bleeding injury).

· All educational and public health departments, regardless of whether AIDS-infected children are involved, are strongly encouraged to inform parents, children, and educators of facts regarding AIDS and its transmission. Such education would greatly assist efforts to provide the best care and education for infected children while minimizing the risk of transmission to others.

142. Are all states instituting the aforementioned recommendations?

These recommendations are guidelines proposed by the CDC and will be evaluated and implemented by each community according to its needs. In New York, where the greatest number of cases of AIDS in school-aged children exists, the New York City health commissioner has set up a committee composed of a parent, medical and educational experts, and a social worker to address each case on an individual basis. The Philadelphia Board of Education recently unanimously voted to allow children with AIDS to attend school with the approval of a special screening committee. Alternately, the recent decision of the San Diego Board of Education to ban students with AIDS from public classrooms, contrary to CDC recommendations, emphasizes the differences in how communities may view and deal with this complex social problem.

143. What steps are public health officials taking in the United States to reduce the spread of AIDS virus infection?

Because the behaviors that spread the AIDS virus are voluntary and occur with mutual consent, public eduction and individual counseling remain the two most appropriate avenues for controlling AIDS virus spread. Programs aimed at emphasizing the dangers of intravenous drug abuse and the risks of sexual contact with members of high risk groups exist in many school systems and seem crucial in reducing the incidence of AIDS infection. Large-scale programs by the American Medical Association and U.S. Public Health Service are currently underway, whereby publications, videotapes, and other educational materials are made accessible to physicians and the general public.

144. What role do public health experts feel quarantining those with AIDS has?

Quarantining refers to the act of imposing restrictions, sometimes geographic, on a person to prevent transmission of an infectious disease to another person. The American College of Physicians and the Infectious Diseases Society of America recently issued a position paper defining policies that support the dissemination of accurate information on AIDS and the reduction of AIDS virus transmission. The position that quarantining persons with AIDS or AIDS viral infection is impractical and medically and ethically unsound was based on the following rationale:

- Quarantining appears to be an unjustified invasion of individual liberty and privacy.
- Quarantining would be counterproductive in that many physicians would be less likely to report cases of AIDS to public health officials. Such failure to report would alter data collection and the cooperation of risk group members, activities important to understanding conditions caused by the AIDS virus.
- A person infected with the AIDS virus but without clinical symptoms is capable of infecting another person. Quarantining those with AIDS is therefore discriminatory. In addition, quarantining those with symptoms is impractical as a means of reducing AIDS virus transmission because it is estimated that the ratio of asymptomatic carriers of the AIDS virus to persons with AIDS is greater than 100:1.
- The quarantining of particular individuals with AIDS or AIDS infection who openly engage in sexual behavior or drug abuse in a manner that threatens others cannot be expected to control an epidemic that is frequently transmitted by asymptomatic persons unaware that they are carriers.
- Quarantining a small group of persons with AIDS would communicate a false sense of security to other infected and high-risk persons who may assume that incarceration of others implies approval to engage in sexual behaviors and drug practices known to transmit the AIDS virus.

145. Is an imployer legally able to terminate employment of a person with AIDS or antibody positivity?

An extensive review on the legality of employment discrimination against persons with AIDS or AIDS virus infection has revealed that no cases have reached an appellate level in any jurisdiction as of 1987.

Because state laws concerning disability discrimination are a relatively recent phenomenon, none specifically addresses AIDS and there appear to be only a few relating to those with "infectious conditions," "illnesses," or "transmissible diseases." Instead, state laws dealing with discrimination in the work setting have focused on the "physically disabled" or "handicapped." Although the federal Rehabilitation Act of 1973 prohibits discrimination against those with a handicap or a perceived handicapping condition in any program receiving federal funding, it does not apply to any employer who does not receive such funding. Most hospitals, public schools, and governmental agencies are covered by the Rehabilitation Act, but private employers are generally not covered by that legislation. Rather, jurisdiction over laws regarding employment discrimination rests with each state. Most states have so far enacted legislation protecting the physically disabled. The different language of each state's laws will ultimately determine if persons with AIDS fit the definition of physically disabled in all cases.

Each of the 50 states and the District of Columbia has either statutory or executive requirements of equal rights for the disabled, although in some jurisdictions (Alabama, Arkansas, Delaware, Idaho, and Mississippi) these apply primarily to government employees. In several states, gubernatorial executive orders or legislative enactments extend the nondiscrimination requirement to programs receiving state financial assistance (Arkansas, Idaho, Mississippi, and Virginia.) In Georgia and Kentucky, discrimination against physically disabled persons is illegal; however, persons with "communicable diseases" are excluded from such protection. In New Hampshire, persons with an "illness" are distinguished from those with a physical disability and are also excluded from discrimination-employment protection laws.

Among the laws protecting the disabled from employment discrimination, the definition of physically handicapped varies greatly. Federal regulations and 13 states broadly define handicapped as "one who has a physical or mental impairment which substantially limits one or more of such person's major life activities." Six states (Alaska, Maine, Maryland, Montana, Nebraska, and New Jersey) currently have variations of a basic definition covering discrimination against those "with an anatomical, physiological or neurological disability, infirmity, malformation, or disfigurement which is caused by injury, birth defect, or illness." California defines physical handicap, in part, as ". . . impairment of physical ability because of . . . loss of function or coordination, or any other health impairment which requires special education or related services." In New York, handicap means "physical . . . impairment resulting from . . . physiological . . . conditions which prevents the exercise of a normal bodily function or is demonstrated by medically accepted clinical or laboratory diagnosis techniques." Four states (Indiana, Kansas, Iowa, and Missouri) merely define physical disability as a condition resulting in substantial disability. Some states (Florida, North Carolina, Virginia, Tennessee, and Nevada) provide no definition of handicap in their statutes protecting against discrimination of physically handicapped in the work environment. Although there have been few reported decisions as to whether AIDS-related medical conditions are covered by these statutes, the human rights commissions in each state have been nearly unanimous in holding such conditions to be covered.

Nearly all laws governing discrimination against physically disabled persons make it legal to terminate a physically disabled person from work if the physical requirements of the job cannot be performed. However, even this criterion has been subject to differing interpretation. Nevertheless, it seems, despite varying language between jurisdictions, that most states appear to protect persons with AIDS or exposure to the AIDS virus from employment discrimination by statutes protecting the physically disabled. In addition, the recognition that AIDS is transmissible in adults through sexual contact and the intravenous sharing of needles suggests that laws that give employers the right to exclude disabled persons from employment if such employment would threaten the health of employees are not applicable to persons with AIDS. The legality of discriminating against a person with AIDS in the work setting ultimately awaits court tests that take into account the specific language of discrimination laws specific to the particular jurisdiction.

146. Has there been any legislative body that has ruled that AIDS is a handicap?

While no state or federal judiciary has yet incorporated AIDS in their statutes or laws related to employment discrimination of the physically handicapped, local jurisdictions have passed or amended their own ordinances defining AIDS as a protected handicap that cannot lawfully be made the basis for employment decisions. Such laws have been passed in Los Angeles, San Francisco, West Hollywood (California), Berkeley (California), Philadelphia, and Hennepin County (Minnesota).

147. Can an employer ask a prospective applicant if he or she has taken an AIDS antibody test?

If the language of a specific federal, state, or local law specifies that AIDS meets the criterion of a handicap or disability, and if the law forbids using disability as a basis for employment decisions, a job applicant cannot be asked if he has had an AIDS antibody test.

148. Can an employer request that employees submit to AIDS antibody testing as part of the company exam?

If AIDS is a protected handicap in the jurisdiction under which the company is located, the antibody test cannot be requested of employees or made part of the routine examinations often required to determine fitness for work. In addition, California and Wisconsin, irrespective of their laws regarding discrimination against the handicapped and disabled, have enacted specific legislation making the communication of the results of an individual's antibody status to anyone other than a health care provider for purposes of direct medical care a criminal offense punishable by fine and/or imprisonment. This law precludes employers in these states from requesting that employees submit to antibody testing.

149. Are there any publications that provide current information and updates on legal issues surrounding AIDS?

The Lambda Legal Defense and Education Fund (LAMBDA) is a national organization that has established and maintained a national clearinghouse for AIDS and the law, including legislation and litigation materials (AIDS Clearinghouse, 666

Brady, 12th Floor, New York, NY 10012, 212-995-8585). It publishes a monthly *AIDS Update*, reviewing AIDS-related legal materials, and the *AIDS Legal Guide*, 2nd edition, available at the same address. *AIDS Policy and Law* is a bi-weekly newsletter also focusing on current policy and litigation surrounding AIDS. It is available for a subscription price of $337 yearly (BNA Publishing, 202-452-7889).

CHAPTER SEVEN

The Epidemiology of AIDS

150. Will reach epidemic proportions?

AIDS has already met the definition of an epidemic, which is a period or outbreak of unusually high incidence of a disease in a community or area. AIDS is already considered a pandemic, which is an epidemic over a wide geographic area, usually worldwide.

151. From what areas of the world have cases of AIDS been reported?

As of December 1986, the World Health Organization had received reports of approximately 35,000 cases of AIDS from 74 countries. The United States has the largest number of cases and the European count was estimated at approximately 3,000.

While data from only 1985 is available for individual countries, the number of AIDS cases has proportionately increased since then for all countries. As of 1985, the highest total number of European cases were from Germany and France, whereas the highest number of European cases per million population were from Belgium, Denmark, and Switzerland.

In North and South America, Haiti, Canada, and Brazil had the largest number of the 778 non-U.S. reported cases, while Haiti, Grenada, and Trinidad had the largest number of cases per million persons. Australia also reported a substantial number of AIDS cases. Cases have been reported from Japan, China, Thailand, Singapore, Saudi Arabia, and Indonesia as well.

In Central Africa alone, in 1985, the annual incidence of AIDS was estimated at from 170 to 400 cases per million population. The estimates of 550 to 1,000 cases per million people annually in Central Africa as of late 1986 emphasize the seriousness of AIDS as a public health dilemma for countries outside of the United States.

152. How does the prevalence of AIDS compare in countries outside of the United States?

The World Health Organization Collaborating Centre on AIDS along with other governmental agencies maintains statistics on AIDS. The number of AIDS cases per million population has steadily increased for each country since the initial tabulation of the data in October 1985, given as follows. These estimates of the prevalence of the disease, which is how the data was first reported by WHO, show the relative severity of the problem that AIDS presents to each country. The prevalence figures are followed by actual numbers of cases reported to WHO by countries that have filed cases up to June 1987. All case numbers are reported by the individual country without independent confirmation and, in most cases, probably underestimate the true number of cases.

Country	Cases of AIDS/Million Population (October 1985)
North and South America	
Haiti	59.7
United States	55.9
Grenada	20
Trinidad	13.3
Canada	6.6
Brazil	1.4
Mexico	0.2
Europe and Other Countries	
Zaire	170–400*

*Estimated at from 550–1,000 as of June 1986.

Belgium	11.9
Switzerland	11.8
Denmark	11.2
France	8.5
Netherlands	5.7
West Germany	4.8
Sweden	4.3
United Kingdom	4.0
Norway	3.3
Austria	3.1
Finland	2.0
Italy	1.6
Spain	1.6
Greece	1.0

Country	Total AIDS Cases in Representative Countries through June 1987
North and South America	
United States	35,980
Brazil	1,695
Canada	1,000
Mexico	407
Argentina	78
Europe and Other Countries	
France	1,632
Uganda	1,138
West Germany	1,089
United Kingdom	791
Rwanda	705
Italy	664
Australia	481
Spain	357
Central African Republic	202
Denmark	150

South Africa	70
Soviet Union	32
India	9

153. Why is the prevalence of AIDS so high in Africa?

Shortly after AIDS was first identified, cases were noted in Africans who were living in Europe. By early 1986, 177 cases of Africans with AIDS had been identified in Europe. The original homes of these persons were traced to 24 different countries, mostly in Central Africa. Unlike the American cases of AIDS that occurred principally in homosexual men and intravenous drug abusers, these African individuals denied homosexuality or drug abuse and the ratio of cases was nearly equal among men and women.

Because of the unexpected number of Africans with AIDS, epidemiological studies were initiated with the purpose of understanding the aforementioned data. These studies showed that the AIDS virus was widely spread throughout Central Africa, with the highest incidence occurring in female prostitutes. Further investigation revealed that clusters of AIDS cases were found to be linked by heterosexual contact.

A review of stored blood showed that antibody to the AIDS virus was easily detectable in some areas of Africa as early as 1963. While retrospective examination of records of those who died from opportunistic infections found individuals as far back as 1975 who would meet the present CDC definition of AIDS, the earliest reported evidence for the presence of the AIDS virus was found in stored serum initially obtained in Kinshasa, Zaire in 1959. Use of antibody testing in Africa to determine the prevalence of the virus has been complicated by malaria, which may interfere with the ELISA test.

It is difficult to know where the virus first entered the human population. What is clear is that large increases in the various opportunistic infections characteristic of AIDS began occurring in Africa in the late 1970s. Because African patients commonly presented with a number of gastrointestinal illnesses, the syndrome of chronic diarrhea, loss of appetite, and marked weight loss common in Uganda and Tanzania became locally known as "slim disease" before AIDS was fully recognized in the United States. It seems that sporadic cases of

AIDS-related illnesses occurred in Africa prior to its recognition in other parts of the world. A small lead time over the United States and an early appearance in the heterosexual population may have given the virus the opportunity to disseminate to its current proportions in Africa.

154. Where does the situation in Africa now stand?

It is very hard to know with any degree of certainty the true scale of the AIDS problem in Africa. Diagnoses may be made in only the most obvious cases because of the cost and lack of sophisticated laboratory tests that are useful in diagnosing many opportunistic infections and AIDS virus exposure. Throughout large areas of Africa, the health services may see only a fraction of the total cases of AIDS because of the unavailability of health care for many people. The case reporting system in the principal cities of Rwanda and Zaire, two of the most severely affected countries, indicates the yearly rate of AIDS cases to be at around 800 per million population and 180 per million population, respectively. Estimates by epidemiologists place the actual incidence much higher, with most projections being around 1,000 per million population per year.

All studies examining the spread of the AIDS virus through Africa show that the rise is rapid and unabated. In Kinshasa, Zaire, examination of the stored blood samples of pregnant women showed that the incidence of antibody positivity rose from 0 to 8 percent over a 16-year period. Clearly, Africa has the potential to have millions of cases of AIDS develop within the next few years. International committees are currently being established to monitor the presence of the AIDS virus and its spread into various populations. It is hoped that improved cooperation between countries will lead to better public health measures and education to slow the virus as it moves into increasingly larger portions of the African population.

The enormous task African countries face in initiating practical social policies to curtail the transmission of the AIDS virus is underscored by the following facts: (1) the $60 million expense to screen blood for the AIDS virus in the United States in 1985 represented an amount in excess of the entire health budget for many African countries, (2) the cost of caring for ten AIDS patients in the United States exceeds the entire annual budget for most large hospitals in Central Africa, and (3) when many hospitals in African countries have limited funds to buy necessary items such as antibiotics, policies emphasizing the need to purchase new needles rather than reuse disposable ones may prove ineffective.

155. Does the pattern of disease in Africa have meaning for AIDS in the United States?

Africa may provide important clues to what lies ahead for AIDS in the Western world. In the West, the major risk groups are homosexual men and intravenous drug abusers. However, in Central Africa where the incidence of AIDS is relatively high, the male-to-female ratio of the disease is approximately equal, and a large number of cases involve heterosexual transmission from male to female and vice versa. Just as the homosexual and intravenous drug abuser patterns of transmission in the United States are serving as predictors for countries such as Australia and Japan which are now reporting their initial surges of AIDS cases among homosexual men, Zaire and other African countries may serve as models for the United States now that the virus has entered the American heterosexual population.

156. If the presence of the AIDS virus or antibody positivity is a necessary criterion to meet the CDC definition of AIDS, how is AIDS diagnosed in underdeveloped countries where AIDS virus detection is unavailable or not widely used?

Adults

AIDS in an adult is defined by the existence of at least two of the following major signs associated with at least one minor sign, in the absence of known causes of immunosuppression such as cancer or preexisting severe malnutrition.

Major Signs

· Weight loss > 1 month

- Chronic diarrhea > 1 month
- Prolonged fever > 1 month, intermittent or constant

Minor Signs

- Persistent cough > 1 month
- Generalized itching and inflammation of the skin
- Recurrent herpes zoster, a typically painful skin disorder characterized by vesicular eruptions
- Oropharyngeal candidiasis, a fungal oral infection
- Chronic progressive and widespread infection with herpes simplex, a virus capable of producing disease of the mouth, skin, eye, brain, and genital tract
- Generalized lymphadenopathy (enlarged lymph nodes)

The presence of Kaposi's sarcoma or cryptococcal meningitis (an inflammation of the lining of the brain due to the fungus Cryptococcus neoformans) is sufficient by itself for a person to be classified as having AIDS.

Children

Pediatric AIDS is suspected in an infant or child presenting with at least two major signs in association with at least two minor signs, in the absence of known causes of immunosuppression.

Major Signs

- Weight loss or abnormally slow growth
- Chronic diarrhea > 1 month
- Prolonged fever > 1 month, intermittent or constant

Minor Signs

- Generalized lymphadenopathy
- Oropharyngeal candidiasis
- Repeated common infections of the middle ear or mouth
- Persistent cough > 1 month
- Generalized inflammation of the skin
- Confirmed infection of mother with AIDS virus

157. Are foreign countries employing measures to combat AIDS?

Other countries have initiated educational programs and public policies to minimize the spread of AIDS. For example, Pakistan has announced that persons who have lived outside the country for more than four years will not be accepted as blood donors. In China, the import of human plasma has been barred. In England, the Public Health Control of Diseases Act was passed by Parliament, which gives public health officials the power to quarantine infected individuals to hospital settings. The association between the first two cases of AIDS reported in Saudi Arabia in 1985 and blood imported from the United States in 1981 has strengthened calls of many countries to limit and screen blood products obtained from the United States.

158. As of March 9, 1987, approximately 32,000 cases of AIDS had been reported to CDC from the United States. What was the geographic distribution of these cases?

By early 1986, cases of AIDS had been reported from all 50 states. As of early 1987, more than 50 percent of all AIDS cases had been reported from New York and California, where the concentrations of risk groups are the greatest. Idaho, Montana, North Dakota, South Dakota, Vermont, and Wyoming had the lowest number of AIDS cases, with less than ten each. As of March 1987, New York City alone accounted for over one-third of all known AIDS cases, and San Francisco accounted for approximately 10 percent of all known cases.

159. What is the incidence of AIDS in Americans not in a known risk group?

The incidence of AIDS for those not in any "risk" group is around one in a million. When data from two separate sources are analyzed, they independently support this estimate:

- The prevalence of antibody positivity in blood donors not in risk groups is around 1 in 10,000. Since studies have estimated that the prevalence of cases of antibody positivity-to-AIDS cases is approximately 100:1 in the general population, the probability of a person with AIDS not being in a known risk group is approximately (1/10,000)/100 or one in a million.

· Of the 29,000 cases reported up to January 1987, 853 or approximately 3 percent did not appear to fit into any major risk group. However, after assessment of factors such as inability to interview the person due to death (158), refusal to be interviewed (206), and those cases still under investigation (458), only 184 persons with AIDS were clearly identified as belonging to no known risk group. Given reports from the CDC that many individuals in this group have had sexual contacts with prostitutes whose antibody status was unknown, the actual number of AIDS cases fitting into no identifiable risk group is probably much lower than estimated. When the entire population of Americans is considered, the prevalence of AIDS cases not in any known risk group approximates one in a million.

160. Are there other statistics that can illuminate the scope of the problem?

Data from death certificates reveal that in 1984, AIDS was among the five leading causes of death in New York City among males aged 25 to 54 years, and the leading cause of death for males age 30 to 39 years. For females, AIDS was the fourth leading cause of death in women in New York City aged 25 to 29 years, and the second leading cause for women aged 30 to 34 years.

Investigators have summarized the effect AIDS has had on life expectancy using "years of potential life lost" as an indicator of premature death before age 65. Using this criterion, AIDS was the fourth leading cause of years of potential life lost among males aged 15 to 64 in 1984 and ranked slightly less than all cancers in years lost in the same age group. Data from more recent death certificates in New York City are still being tabulated and estimates are that for 1985 AIDS will have been the leading cause of years of potential life lost among males aged 15 to 64 years, surpassing homicides-suicides, heart disease, and cancer.

161. What is predicted regarding the future growth of AIDS in the United States?

In November 1986, the U.S. Public Health Service estimated that about 250,000 new cases of AIDS will occur by 1991 and approximately 180,000 deaths will have occurred within the decade after the disease was first recognized. These projections were based upon the current number of AIDS cases and the fact that most of those who will have symptoms of AIDS in the next five years are presently infected with the virus. Between January 1987 and January 1988, it is estimated that over 30,000 new cases of AIDS will occur. While it is difficult to estimate the future incidence of AIDS, a number of statistics demonstrates the gravity of the problem:

- The Surgeon General of the United States estimates that in the year 1991, an estimated 145,000 persons with AIDS will need health and supportive services at a total cost of from $8 to 16 billion.
- In the United States, the number of new cases of persons with AIDS was 747 in 1982, 2,124 in 1983, 4,569 in 1984, 8,406 in 1985, and 15,200 in 1986.
- As of March 1987, the number of persons with AIDS appeared to be doubling every 11 monhs.
- It is estimated that there are presently 1 to 1.5 million people in the United States infected with the AIDS virus. Epidemiological studies suggest that approximately 20 to 30 percent of these individuals will develop AIDS or an AIDS-related illness within the next five years.
- The World Health Organization predicts, based on current trends, that the number of people infected by the AIDS virus worldwide could reach 100 million by the end of this decade.

162. What are the economic costs of AIDS in the United States?

Because of the recurrent, prolonged infections and the debilitating nature of the disease, the cost of treatment for AIDS patients is among the most expensive of all disease treatments. The economic impact of the first 10,000 persons with AIDS is profound. These patients averaged 166 total hospital days at an estimated cost of $140,000 per patient. They also lost an average of 360 work days and $19,000 in income during the time of their illness. Future earnings lost to premature death approach $460,000 per patient. Thus, for the first 10,000 persons with AIDS, it is estimated that the total economic impact of their illness was approximately $6.3 billion, with $1.4 billion of that total attributed to direct medical costs.

In 1985, the average lifespan of persons with AIDS was estimated to be 224 days after hospitalization for the first opportunistic infection. Of that time, patients were hospitalized an average of 160 days. Using a conservative estimate of $100,000 for the average direct lifetime hospital cost of an AIDS patient, the expense for the additional 16,000 cases of AIDS expected in 1986 will be approximately $1.6 billion. This figure does not include the additional costs of outpatient care, medication, lost employment, reduced productivity, shortened life expectancy, social welfare services, and antibody testing of all blood donations.

In the fall of 1985, the average daily cost for treating an AIDS patient was about $800. This figure was more than 60 percent higher than the cost of treating other patients, and approximately $300 of this daily bill was left unpaid. Because New York City provides financial coverage for those patients without insurance, it is estimated that the annual bill for this purpose was approximately $45 million. In Los Angeles alone, the average cost of one hospitalization for an AIDS patient is more than three times the average cost for hospitalizing a non-AIDS patient. Of this bill, approximately 35 percent is left unpaid and is absorbed by the hospital. At a time when some states are enacting legislation to provide cost containment for health care, the rapidly rising cost of AIDS care will pose serious challenges to efforts to limit growing health costs.

163. Are there acceptable sites less costly than hospitals to care for AIDS patients?

A recent study sought to better understand the ways in which those with AIDS utilize hospital resources. It was found that 15 percent of 273 patients were able to leave the hospital at least once during the late stages of their illness when they had a spouse, friend, or family member willing to accommodate their needs. In contrast, the unavailability of family members and friends to care for many homeless AIDS patients and the lack of organized community health services are believed to result in longer and more costly hospitalizations than might be medically necessary. Consequently, financial and educational support have been proposed for hospital-affiliated outpatient programs and home-care settings for AIDS patients. The presence of community health services for AIDS patients in San Francisco is credited for the low cost of hospital care there, which averages approximately $29,000 per AIDS patient or $118,000 below the national average.

The Robert Wood Johnson Foundation announced in March 1986 the availability of $17.2 million to ten cities for the development of outpatient health care, in-home health care and counseling, and hospice services for AIDS patients medically able to leave the hospital setting. Despite these early efforts, it is clear that much remains to be done to facilitate extending compassionate, quality medical care to the home. The projected hospital costs of caring for increasing numbers of AIDS patients make alternate care facilities critical to cost containment.

CHAPTER EIGHT

Research and Funding for AIDS

164. How much money is being appropriated for AIDS research?

Congress budgeted $416 million during fiscal year 1987 to combat AIDS and recently received the Administration's fiscal year 1988 budget requesting $534 million. These figures represent dramatic increases from the $5.5 million initially allocated in fiscal year 1982 and the $234 million more recently allocated for fiscal year 1986. The money scheduled by Congress for AIDS research in fiscal year 1987 is approximately 5 percent of the total amount appropriated to the National Institutes of Health. Until 1986, both the National Institutes of Health and the CDC had supported AIDS research, in part, by redirecting funds originally targeted for research on other diseases. A joint study by the National Institute of Medicine and the National Academy of Sciences, released in November 1986, predicted that at least $2 billion per year will be required to combat AIDS by 1990. It recommended an increase in funds from about $400 million scheduled by Congress during fiscal year 1987 to approximately $1 billion per year by 1990.

165. Where will the $534 million requested for fiscal year 1988 go?

Of the $534 million requested for AIDS in fiscal year 1988, about $121 million is targeted for educational efforts, $185 million is scheduled to support basic research, and $228 million is for the development of treatments for AIDS.

A variety of governmental agencies will be awarded these funds and will be responsible for distributing monies to academic centers and other agencies. The CDC will direct a large proportion of its funds for educational and risk-reduction programs through grants to state and local organizations and to continued work toward the development of a vaccine. In addition to conducting their own research through National Institutes of Health-based scientists, the National Institutes of Health will award a large proportion of its funds to researchers at academic institutions to conduct laboratory and clinical investigations. The clinical testing of a variety of experimental antiviral agents will also continue at the National Institutes of Health and selected institutions. Many governmental agencies will be involved in funding information services and counseling for both persons with AIDS and care providers, as well as funding public education programs emphasizing means to reduce the risk of virus transmission.

166. How does the $264 million appropriated for AIDS research in fiscal year 1986 compare with money appropriated for other medical research?

Of the $965 billion federal budget for fiscal year 1986, $5.13 billion was scheduled for the National Institutes of Health. Appropriations targeted for major divisions within the National Institutes of Health include:

National Cancer Institute: $1.126 billion, of which $926 million was targeted for cancer research

National Heart, Lung, and Blood Institute: $733 million for research into heart and related disorders

National Institute of Neurological and Communicative Disorders: $360 million for research into strokes, multiple sclerosis, dementia, and other diseases of the nervous system

National Institues of Allergy and Infectious Diseases: $340 million for research into transmissible diseases and disorders of the immune system

167. Are there any experimental drugs currently being tested against the AIDS virus?

There are several experimental drugs, including suramin, ribavirin, HPA-23, AL 721, and azidothymidine (AZT), currently under investigation as antiviral agents. In late 1985, the National Cancer Institute initiated clinical trials with seven other institutions to evaluate suramin. In several cases, suppressed reproduction of the virus was achieved but no long-term clinical benefit was shown. Preliminary laboratory research with the four other drugs, ribivarin, AZT, AL 721, and HPA-23, has also shown these agents to be capable of inhibiting reproduction of the AIDS virus in lymphocytes. Clinical trials evaluating these drugs are currently underway at the National Institutes of Health and a variety of academic institutions, including New York University-Cornell Medical Center, the Universities of California at San Francisco and Los Angeles, Duke Medical Center, and the Memorial Sloan-Kettering Cancer Center in New York.

While preliminary research has shown that these drugs could limit the multiplication of the AIDS virus, and that the use of AZT could result in short-term clinical and immunological improvement in some patients, the drugs have not altered the progression of the disease nor the survival rate of persons with AIDS. Of the drugs mentioned here, only AZT can leave the blood and enter into the brain. This is a critical feature in the design of an antiviral drug that is to be effective against a virus that infects cells residing in the brain and spinal cord.

168. What are the short-term clinical and immunological improvements that have occurred in some patients given AZT?

In September 1986, preliminary trials revealed that only one of 145 patients receiving AZT had died in the same period in which 16 of 137 patients receiving placebo had died. Based on these results in certain patients with AIDS, the FDA is allowing the manufacturer of AZT, Burroughs Wellcome Company, to bypass certain normal institutional review procedures and increase the availability of AZT to selected persons. While no improved long-term survival or reversal or immunological abnormalities has been demonstrated with AZT, it was felt that the study results warranted greater availability of AZT prior to the standard evaluation given all drugs. However, patients eligible for AZT must meet certain criteria and must have sufficiently advanced disease to warrant therapy with a drug that may have immediate, unknown side effects. Studies with AZT in HIV-infected patients are ongoing. Because of the rapidly evolving information about the drug and its utility in patients, a national hot line at the NIH, providing updated information on AZT for both physicians and other individuals, has been established. Information can be obtained by calling 800-843-9388.

169. What is the experimental drug previously used by AIDS patients in France?

This is the antiviral drug HPA-23 mentioned previously, currently approved for experimental use in the United States and under evaluation at a number of medical centers.

170. Are there any clues as to how some experimental drugs limit the multiplication of the AIDS virus in lymphocyte cells?

Yes. The AIDS virus is composed of a protein coat and an inner core of the nucleic acid RNA. When the virus infects a cell, it must use an enzyme called reverse transcriptase to set up a chain of events which allow it to use its own RNA to produce the nucleic acid, DNA. This newly created DNA is necessary to allow the multiplication of the AIDS virus through which other cells are infected and killed. Some of the aforementioned experimental drugs have been shown to interfere with the ability of reverse transcriptase to properly form DNA from the RNA of the virus. While there remains a large gap between this finding and demonstrating a clinical benefit to persons with AIDS, it is an important step in the process of developing curative drugs.

171. Can the body ever spontaneously rid itself of the AIDS virus without the use of drugs?

In animals, retroviruses appear to remain indefinitely or until death of the infected host. In humans, the AIDS virus has been isolated years after the onset of any of the AIDS virus syndromes, including antibody positivity. The virus seems to become an integral part of the infected cell and is passed on with the cell as it divides in the living host. Without destroying all the infected cells, it seems unlikely that the virus can be eliminated spontaneously or even with the use of drugs.

172. Are there any other developments that might accelerate AIDS research?

The finding of Simian Acquired Immunodeficiency Syndrome (SAIDS) in macaque monkeys has not only given clues to the origin of AIDS but may also provide a useful model to study the natural history of the disease and help in the development of effective antiviral drugs. In the African Green monkey, the presence of a retrovirus similar to the AIDS virus that infects in the absence of disease may provide vital information helpful to the development of a vaccine. Additionally, several structural components of the AIDS virus necessary both for virus replication and destruction of the infected T-lymphocyte were identified in early 1986. This discovery holds promise for future work in the development of new therapies for AIDS.

173. Isn't the Food and Drug Administration "dragging its foot" in approving drugs for experimental use in AIDS patients?

The FDA granted approval for HPA-23 to be used as an investigational drug within five days of receiving application from Rhone-Poulenc pharmaceutical manufacturers. Within a short period of time, five academic centers had been awarded funding to initiate studies with AIDS patients.

AZT was approved for limited human testing less than one week after application by investigators. When preliminary results revealed short-term benefits of AZT in selected AIDS patients, the FDA by-passed certain institutional drug review procedures to allow its manufacturer to make AZT available on a "humane, compassionate" basis to selected patients.

174. What are the steps a drug must go through before being approved for experimental use and eventually having its designation changed from experimental to approved?

Medical history is full of anecdotal claims of the effectiveness of treatments for a wide range of diseases and illnesses, claims that have often not stood the test of time and rigorous scientific evaluation. The responsibility to evaluate the effectiveness and safety of drugs before approving them for use rests with the FDA. The process of drug approval is done in a series of steps. Initially, a manufacturer will apply for permission to clinically evaluate a drug in a specified setting. Permission to grant the use of a drug in this limited experimental setting is based on data from prior animal or other laboratory research and on the evaluation of the risks and benefits of the drug to the individuals in the proposed study.

Participants in these studies are fully informed of the known risks and benefits of the therapy. If approved for experimental use, Phase I trials begin with the initial introduction of the drug into humans with special attention paid to any short-term side effects. Phase II trials are conducted on patient volunteers and are designed to expand the inquiry of Phase I trials. There is sometimes a comparison group of volunteers not receiving the drug but instead a placebo. Phase III trials are conducted on hundreds of patients with proper control groups, and involve prolonged observation to determine the drug's effectiveness. Because of the uniform deadlines of AIDS, the unavailability of effective treatments, and the judgment that side effects of many experimental drugs are outweighed by the devastating effects of the disease, antiviral agents to be tested against AIDS are beginning Phase III testing in a remarkably short time.

175. Where is AIDS research being done?

Research on potential treatment for AIDS is focused on three modalities: the development of antiviral therapies to inhibit the reproduction of the virus, medications that may strengthen the immune response, and medications designed to better fight opportunistic infection. Laboratory research is being done at a variety of institutions including the National Institutes of

Health, the Pasteur Institute in Paris, and several major American universities. Most epidemiological data are being tabulated by the CDC. Clinical studies are being performed at many hospitals, particularly in areas where the AIDS epidemic has been centered.

In light of new projections that the number of new cases of AIDS will be increasing dramatically over the next five years, the National Institutes of Health has funded 14 major medical centers $20 million per year for five years to test the application of newly developed therapies for persons with AIDS. These centers are Harvard University, Boston; The Johns Hopkins Medical Institutions, Baltimore; Memorial Sloan-Kettering Cancer Center, New York City; New York University, New York City; Stanford University, Palo Alto, California; University of California at Los Angeles; University of California at San Diego; University of California at San Francisco; University of Miami, Florida; University of Pittsburgh; University of Rochester, New York; University of Southern California, Los Angeles; University of Texas and the M.D. Anderson Hospital and Tumor Institute, Houston; and the University of Washington, Seattle.

176. Are any private philanthropic foundations involved in funding for AIDS research?

Private foundations are participating in combatting AIDS. A national research foundation, the American Foundation for AIDS Research (AMFAR), was formed in 1985 by the merger of the AIDS Medical Foundation in New York and the National AIDS Research Foundation of Los Angeles. The primary purpose of AMFAR is to use private donations to fund research geared toward a better understanding of AIDS transmission and treatment.

177. Where can money for patient care and research on AIDS be donated?

AMFAR is a nonprofit organization that accepts donations. It has two main offices, located at 9601 Wilshire Boulevard, Mezzanine, Los Angeles, CA 90210 (213-273-5547) and 40

West 57th Street, Suite 406, New York, NY 10019 (212-333-3118). The Elisabeth Kubler-Ross Center (South Route 616, Head Waters, VA 24442, 703-396-3441) is another nonprofit organization and provides workshops and care for many persons with AIDS, particularly children. Since persons with AIDS are not charged, their financial ability to receive this care is based solely on private donations. Donations to both of the above organizations may be tax-deductible.

In addition, local agencies providing AIDS information may be able to direct individuals more specifically to particular foundations or organizations applicable to the donor's interests.

178. Are there any federal assistance programs for which a person with AIDS is eligible and to which he can directly apply?

The Social Security Administration administers two programs for which persons with AIDS may be eligible: the Supplemental Security Income (SSI) program, in which assistance is based on the medical condition and financial status of the applicant, and the Social Security Disability (SSD) program, in which assistance is based on medical condition and employment history. Since disability is defined by both programs as any illness preventing or expected to prevent a person from working at least 12 months, many persons with AIDS or AIDS-related illnesses may meet these eligibility criteria.

CHAPTER NINE

Resource Centers for AIDS Information and Support

179. What groups offer information on AIDS for the general public? How about support for persons with AIDS or AIDS-related illnesses?

The Office of the Surgeon General of the United States and the Medical News Departments of the *Journal of the American Medical Association* and *Occupational Health and Safety* have independently compiled a list of resource centers, both national and local, along with hot lines and other services that provide information to members of high risk groups for AIDS. Most of these centers also provide educational materials for anyone interested in acquiring more knowledge about AIDS.

NATIONAL

Centers for Disease Control
Hot line for general information: (800) 342-AIDS
In Atlanta: (404) 329-3524

National Institute of Allergy and Infectious Diseases
Office of Research Reporting and Public Response
(301) 496-5717

AIDS Action Council
Federation of AIDS-Related Organizations
729 Eighth Street, SE
Washington, DC 20003
(202) 547-3101

American Association of Physicians for Human Rights
P.O. Box 14366
San Francisco, CA 94119
(415) 558-9353
In the Bay Area: (415) 673-3189

American Red Cross AIDS Education Office
431 18th Street, NW
Washington, DC 20006
(202) 737-8300

Gay Men's Health Crisis
P.O. Box 274
132 West 24th Street
New York, NY 10011
(212) 807-6655

Hispanic AIDS Forum
c/o APRED
835 Broadway, Suite 2007
New York, NY 10003
(212) 870-1902 or 870-1864

Lambda Legal Defense and Education Fund
666 Broadway, 12th Floor
New York, NY 10012
(212) 995-8585

National AIDS Network
1012 14th Street, NW, Suite 601
Washington, DC 20005
(202) 347-0390

National Coalition of Gay STD Services
P.O. Box 239
Milwaukee, WI 53201

National Gay and Lesbian Task Force
1517 U Street, NW
Washington, DC 20009
(202) 332-6483

National Hemophilia Foundation
Soho Building
110 Greene Street, Room 406
New York, NY 10012
(212) 219-8180

National Lawyers Guild AIDS Network
211 Gough Street, Suite 311
San Francisco, CA 94102
(415) 861-8884

National Lesbian and Gay Health Foundation
P.O. Box 65472
Washington, DC 20035
(202) 797-3708

National Sexually Transmitted Diseases Hotline
American Social Health Association
(800) 227-8922

United States Public Health Service
Hubert Humphrey Building, Room 721-H
200 Independence Avenue, SW
Washington, DC 20201
(202) 245-6867

LOCAL

Arizona

Phoenix

Arizona Stop AIDS Project
736 East Flynn Lane
Phoenix, AZ 85014

Tucson

Tucson Alternative Lifestyle Health Association
101W. Irvington Road, Room B2
Tucson, AZ 85714

Tucson AIDS Project
80 W. Cashing Street
Tucson, AZ 85701
(602) 792-3772

California

Berkeley

Gay Men's Health Collective
2339 Durant Avenue
Berkeley, CA 94704-1670
(415) 644-0425

Pacific Center for Human Growth
2712 Telegraph Avenue
Berkeley, CA 94705
(415) 841-6224

Garden Grove

AIDS Response Program
Gay and Lesbian Community Services Center of Orange County
12832 Garden Grove Boulevard, Suite E
Garden Grove, CA 92643
(714) 534-0862
Hotline: (714) 859-6482

Long Beach

Long Beach Project Ahead
2017 E. 4th Street
Long Beach, CA 90804
(213) 439-3948

Long Beach Department of Health
2655 Pine Avenue
Long Beach, CA 90806
(213) 427-7421

Los Angeles

Aid for AIDS
8235 Santa Monica Boulevard, Suite 311

West Hollywood, CA 90046
(213) 656-1107

AIDS Project/LA
7362 Santa Monica Boulevard
West Hollywood, CA 90046
(213) 876-8951
Hotlines: (213) 876-AIDS and
(800) 992-AIDS (Southern California only)

People with AIDS-LA
c/o Trainor
1752 N. Fuller
Los Angeles, CA 90046

Southern California Mobilization Against AIDS
1428 N. McCadden Place
Los Angeles, CA 90028
(213) 463-3928

Sacramento

California Department of Health Services
AIDS Activities
1812 14th Street, Room 200
Sacramento, CA 95814
(916) 445-0553

Sacramento AIDS/KS Foundation
1900 K Street, Suite 201
Sacramento, CA 95814
(916) 488-AIDS

San Diego

San Diego AIDS Project
P.O. Box 89049
San Diego, CA 92138
(619) 543-0300

Owen Clinic
University of California Medical Center
225 Dickinson Street

San Diego, CA 92103
(619) 543-3995

Beach Area Community Clinic
3705 Mission Boulevard
San Diego, CA 92109
(619) 488-0644

San Francisco

AIDS InterFaith Network
2261 Market Street, #502
San Francisco, CA 94114
(415) 928-4673

AIDS Worried Well Group, Operation Concern
1853 Market Street
San Francisco, CA 94103

Lesbian and Gay Health Services Coordinating Committee
Department of Public Health
101 Grove
San Francisco, CA 94102
(415) 558-2541

People with AIDS/SF
(415) 861-7309

San Francisco AIDS Foundation
333 Valencia Street, Fourth Floor
San Francisco, CA 94103
(415) 864-4376 or 863-2437
Hotline: (800) 367-2437

Shanti Project
525 Howard Street
San Francisco, CA 94105
(415) 777-2273

San Jose

AIDS Hotline: (800) 342-2437

Colorado

Denver

Colorado AIDS Project
P.O. Box 18539
Denver, CO 80218
(303) 837-0166

Connecticut

Hartford

AIDS Coordinator
State Department of Health Services
150 Washington Street
Hartford, CT 06106
(203) 566-1157

New Haven

AIDS Project/New Haven
P.O. Box 636
New Haven, CT 06503
(203) 624-2437

District of Columbia

Whitman-Walker Clinic
1407 S Street
Washington, DC 20009
(202) 332-2437

St. Francis Center
2417 Sherier Place, NW
Washington, DC 20016
(202) 363-8500

Florida

Key West

AIDS Action Committee
201 B Duval Street

Key West, FL 33040
(305) 294-8302

Tampa

Tampa Bay AIDS
P.O. Box 350217
Tampa Bay, FL 33695-0217

Ft. Lauderdale

Health Crisis Network
(305) 674-7530

Miami

Health Crisis Network
P.O. Box 52-1546
Miami, FL 33152
(305) 634-4636

Georgia

Atlanta

AIDS Atlanta
(404) 876-9944

Hawaii

Honolulu

Life Foundation
320 Ward Avenue, Suite 104
Honolulu, HI 96814
(808) 537-2211

Illinois

Chicago

AIDS Action Project
Howard Brown Memorial Clinic
2676 N. Halsted
Chicago, IL 60614
(312) 871-5777

People with AIDS-Chicago
c/o Hall
3414 N. Halsted Street
Chicago, IL 60657

Sable/Sherer Clinic
Fantus Health Center of Cook County Hospital
1835 W. Harrison
Chicago, IL 60612
(312) 633-7810

Kentucky

Lexington

Lexington Gay Services Organization
P.O. Box 11471
Lexington, KY 40511
(606) 231-0335

Maryland

Baltimore

Gay Community Center of Baltimore Health Clinic
241 W. Chase Street, Third Floor
Baltimore, MD 21201
(301) 837-2050

Massachusetts

Boston

Fenway Community Health Center
AIDS Action Committee
16 Haviland Street
Boston, MA 02215
(617) 267-7573

Mayor's Task Force on AIDS
City Hall, Room 608
Boston, MA 02201

Dorchester

Haitian Committee on AIDS in Massachusetts
117 Harvard Street
Dorchester, MA 02124

Michigan

Detroit

Venereal Disease Action Coalition
United Community Services
51 W. Warren Avenue
Detroit, MI 48201
(313) 833-0622

Royal Oak

Wellness Networks Inc.
P.O. Box 1046
Royal Oak, MI 48068
(800) 521-7946, ext. 3582
In Michigan: (800) 482-2404, ext. 3582

Minnesota

Minneapolis

Minnesota AIDS Project
1436 W. Lake Street
Minneapolis, MN 55408
(612) 824-1772

Missouri

St. Louis

AIDS Task Force
c/o Department of Anthropology
Washington University
St. Louis, MO 63130

Nevada

Las Vegas

Southern Nevada Social Services
P.O. Box 71014

Las Vegas, NV 89109
(702) 733-9990

New Jersey

New Brunswick

New Jersey Lesbian and Gay Coalition
P.O. Box 1431
New Brunswick, NJ 08903

Trenton

AIDS Office
New Jersey Department of Health
Health and Agriculture Building
Trenton, NJ 08625
(609) 633-2751

New Mexico

Albuquerque

Common Bond
P.O. Box 1191
Albuquerque, NM 87131
(505) 266-8041

Espanola

New Mexico Physicians for Human Rights
P.O. Box 1361
Espanola, NM 87532

Santa Fe

AIDS Task Force
P.O. Box 968
Santa Fe, NM 87504

New York

Buffalo

Buffalo AIDS Task Force
P.O. Box 38

Bidwell Station
Buffalo, NY 14222
(716) 886-1274

New York City

AIDS Resource Center
24 W. 30th Street, 10th Floor
New York, NY 10001
(212) 481-1270

Gay Men's Health Crisis
Box 274
132 W. 24th Street
New York, NY 10011
(212) 807-6655

New York State AIDS Institute
(212) 340-3388

Community Health Project
208 W. 13th Street
New York, NY 10011
(212) 675-3559

People with AIDS Coalition
263 W. 19th Street
Box 125
New York, NY 10011
(212) 627-1810

Rochester

AIDS Rochester
1063 East Main Street
Rochester, NY 14608

Stony Brook

Long Island AIDS Task Force
SUNY
Stony Brook, NY 11794
(516) 385-2437

White Plains

Mid-Hudson AIDS Task Force
Gay Men's Alliance
255 Grove Street
White Plains, NY 10601

North Carolina

Durham

AIDS Project
Lesbian and Gay Health Project
P.O. Box 11013
Durham, NC 27703
(919) 683-2182

Wilmington

GROW, A Community Service Corp.
P.O. Box 4535
Wilmington, NC 28406
(919) 675-9222

Ohio

Cincinnati

Ambrose Clement Health Clinic
3101 Burnet Avenue
Cincinnati, OH 45229

Columbus

Open Door Clinic
237 E. 17th Street
Columbus, OH 43201
(614) 294-6337

Oregon

Portland

Cascade AIDS Project
408 SW 2nd Avenue

Portland, OR 97204
(503) 223-8299

Texas

Dallas

AIDS Task Force, Dallas Gay Alliance
P.O. Box 190712
Dallas, TX 75219
(214) 528-4233

Houston

KS/AIDS Foundation
3317 Montrose, Box 1155
Houston, TX 77006
(713) 524-AIDS

Utah

Hotline: (303) 831-6268

Virginia

Richmond

Richmond AIDS Information Network
Fan Free Clinic
1721 Hanover Avenue
Richmond, VA 23220
(804) 358-6343

Headwaters

The Elisabeth Kubler-Ross Center
South Route 616
Headwaters, VA 24442
(703) 396-3441

Washington

Seattle

Northwest AIDS Foundation
P.O. Box 3449

Seattle, WA 98114
(206) 587-0306

Seattle AIDS Support
(206) 322-AIDS

AIDS Information Line
Seattle-King County Department of Public Health
(206) 587-4999

Wisconsin

Milwaukee

Brady East STD Clinic
Milwaukee AIDS Project
1240 E. Brady Street
Milwaukee, WI 53202
(414) 272-2144

CANADA

AIDS Committee Toronto (ACT)
P.O. Box 55, Station F
Toronto, M4Y 2L4 Ontario, Canada
(416) 926-1626

180. Where do physicians report newly diagnosed cases of AIDS?

AIDS cases are reported to the Department of Public Health of the respective state. Each Department of Health then reports to the CDC. As of early 1987, nearly all states required that cases of AIDS be reported. In Montana, Tennessee, and American Samoa, reporting is still made on a voluntary basis. AIDS-related illnesses such as ARC or GLS are not reported to the CDC at the present time.

181. Where can free pamphlets that provide information on AIDS be obtained?

The U.S. Public Health Service and the American Red Cross have compiled literature providing *basic* AIDS information. This literature is available at no cost and, although brief, provides accurate, general information focusing on the means of transmission of the AIDS virus.

Leaflets

The following (up to 50 copies) may be obtained by writing AIDS, Suite 700, 1555 Wilson Boulevard, Rosslyn, VA 22209:

"AIDS, Sex and You"
"Facts About AIDS and Drug Abuse"
"AIDS and Your Job—Are There Risks?"
"Gay and Bisexual Men and AIDS"
"AIDS and Children—Information for Parents of School Age Children"
"AIDS and Children—Information for Teachers and School Officials"
"Caring for the AIDS Patient at Home"
"If Your Test for Antibody Positivity to the AIDS Virus is Positive . . . ."

Other Materials Free of Charge

Surgeon General's Report on AIDS (October 1986). Write to AIDS, P.O. Box 14252, Washington, DC 20044 (up to 50 free copies)

Facts About AIDS. Write to AIDS, Suite 700, 1555 Wilson Boulevard, Rosslyn, VA 22209 (up to 50 free copies)

Write to Office of Public Inquiries, Centers for Disease Control, Building 1, Room B-63, 1600 Clifton Road, Atlanta GA 30333 for the following (up to 50 free pamphlets):

"What Everyone Should Know About AIDS" (also available in Spanish)
"Why You Should Be Informed About AIDS" (for health care workers)
"What Gay and Bisexual Men Should Know About AIDS"
"AIDS and Shooting Drugs"

182. Which scientific journals can be examined for up-to-date information on AIDS?

Morbidity and Mortality Weekly Report is published weekly by the CDC/U.S. Public Health Service. It contains ongoing epidemiological information on the number of new AIDS cases reported, and it states recommendations for the prevention of infection. Additionally, the *Journal of the American Medical Association, Lancet, Nature, The New England Journal of Medicine,* and *Science* are weekly publications in which significant basic science and clinical advances concerning AIDS are most likely to be reported.

183. Are there sources for obtaining up-to-date bibliographies of scientific publications on AIDS?

Index Medicus is published monthly by the National Institutes of Health/National Library of Medicine (Superintendent of Documents, U.S. Government Printing Office, Washington, DC 20402) and lists current AIDS-related published scientific articles under the heading ACQUIRED IMMUNE DEFICIENCY SYNDROME. An individual yearly subscription is $161.

Current Contents is a weekly publication that contains the title pages and table of contents of all current scientific journals. This publication has three separate weekly editions pertinent to AIDS (*Clinical Practice, Life Sciences,* and *Social & Behavioral Sciences*) and cross-references AIDS-related articles in the index. It is available from the Institute for Scientific Information, 3501 Market Street, Philadelphia, PA 19104, (800) 523-1850. An individual yearly subscription is $283.

ASCATOPICS® is a weekly publication offered through the Institute for Scientific Information which lists the AIDS-related articles appearing in *Current Contents* (800) 523-1850, ext. 1453. An individual yearly subscription is $175.

    The first two publications are available in all medical school libraries and most hospital libraries.

CHAPTER TEN

Epilogue

184. What are some of the ethical and social dilemmas that the AIDS epidemic has raised?

AIDS has created enormous social and ethical dilemmas that defy simple solutions. The financial burden that AIDS has placed on the health care system has made funding quality patient care even more difficult than before. At a time when funds for scientific research are proportionately decreasing in the yearly federal budget, the proper funding of AIDS research and education is a controversial problem.

The public good must be weighed against the rights of individuals. Confidentiality of antibody positive test results and the access of insurance companies, the military, and the federal government to those results is a social problem of great importance.

Issues involving employment and housing discrimination, liability for cases of AIDS from blood transfusions, and the obligation of infected persons to inform intimate contacts of their infected state are unresolved.

AIDS is a prolonged illness that involves great suffering for patients, friends, and families. How medically aggressive a physician should be for a dying patient and how to help patients decide in advance to undergo life sustaining interventions must be addressed by physician and patient together. The ethical dilemma of what constitutes the best care of the terminally ill person is a problem within medicine which has been heightened by the AIDS crisis.

185. How can medical ethicists help us address these questions?

Answers to ethical questions reflect specific values, prejudices, assumptions, and knowledge of current information

Ethicists can often help reveal the many factors that may underlie and play a part in an individual's ethical decision. While it is clear that no easy answers to the aforementioned questions exist, five rules have been proposed by several ethicists as the basis for dealing with the threats that AIDS allegedly poses to individuals or to society as a whole. These rules are:

- Any alleged threat to the public safety must be both serious and verifiable.
- The means whereby the threat will occur must be specific and recognizable.
- The threat must be absolutely identifiable and not based on suspicion.
- Any imposed restrictions must be known to be effective in containing the threat.
- Words used to define AIDS, such as *serious, verifiable,* and *effective,* must be supported with empirical information and scientific data.

186. What attitudes have Americans developed toward issues of AIDS?

About 51 percent of Americans favored quarantine of those with AIDS, in a December 1985 *Los Angeles Times* poll. The same percentage also favored a law making it a crime for a person with AIDS to have sex with another person. Initiation of laws permitting preemployment screening for AIDS antibodies were supported by 45 percent of those polled, although 51 percent favored laws to protect homosexuals from employment discrimination. Over 50 percent said they would allow their child to attend school in the same classroom as another child with AIDS. In a survey conducted by the American Association of Blood Banks, more than one-third of Americans falsely believed they could acquire AIDS from blood donation, and fewer than half surveyed were aware of antibody testing used by blood banks to screen donated blood for the AIDS virus.

It is clear that Americans have often formed their attitudes about AIDS unaware of information important to the issues at hand. Data from a survey of San Francisco high school students contained in a report by the Institute of Medicine and the National Academy of Sciences in late 1986 emphasized the need for extensive educational programs about the AIDS epidemic. The survey found that approximately 40 percent of the students said they were unaware that AIDS is caused by a virus, one-third thought the disease is casually transmitted, and 40 percent did not know that the use of a condom during sexual intercourse is believed to decrease the risk of infection.

187. What is known about the preferences of those with AIDS to undergo life-sustaining treatments?

Ongoing discussions between those with a terminal illness and their physician concerning life-sustaining procedures (such as cardiopulmonary resuscitation or mechanical ventilation) and certain invasive medical treatments often occur. These discussions are advantageous in that the patient's desires regarding degrees of medical aggressiveness and intervention are known before he becomes too ill to communicate them. Recently, 118 nonhospitalized persons with AIDS were asked:

Had they thought about life-sustaining treatment?
Seventy-eight percent thought a lot or a moderate amount about what care they would want if they developed *Pneumycystis carinii* pneumonia. Sixty-six percent thought a lot or a moderate amount about who they would like to designate to make medical decisions for them if they became unable to do so themselves.

What were their preferences about such treatment?
Ninety-five percent wanted hospitalization and treatment for pneumonia, while only 55 percent wanted admission to the Intensive Care Unit and mechanical ventilation, if medically indicated. If they had *Pneumocystis carinii* pneumonia and were mentally disabled as manifested by severe memory loss, only 19 percent wanted admission to the Intensive Care Unit with mechanical ventilation, and only 17 percent wanted cardiopulmonary resuscitation in the event of a cardiopulmonary arrest.

How did they react to thinking about life-sustaining treatment?

There was a wide variety of different reactions to this question. As a whole, the group was receptive to considering this issue and participating in decision-making about their health care.

What were their preferences for discussing life-sustaining treatment with physicians?

Despite the fact that 73 percent said they wanted to discuss life-sustaining treatment with their physician, only a third had done so. Of those who had these discussions, 58 percent felt the patient should initiate the discussion and 36 percent felt the physician should do so. Responses concerning when such discussions should take place varied and were not limited to a single time for each person. Twenty-four percent wanted to discuss life-sustaining treatment at the time when AIDS was diagnosed, 69 percent wanted such discussions to take place outside the hospital setting before they were seriously ill, 37 percent wanted them on hospital admission, and 54 percent wanted these discussions to occur in the hospital when seriously ill.

Were those with AIDS providing advanced directives to guide care?

Forty-seven percent of persons with AIDS wanted their partners to act as decision-makers concerning life-sustaining treatments if they became mentally incompetent, 32 percent wanted family members, and 14 percent wanted physicians to make the decisions. About two-thirds of the group had provided instructions to their physicians in the event they became mentally incompetent. Twenty-eight percent of the group had initiated a durable power of attorney for health care. This person serves as a legally designated individual who could participate with the physician in medical decision-making if the person with AIDS became unable to do so himself.

188. When a physician finds he or she no longer has any pharmacological treatment for an AIDS patient, what should the physician's responsibility then be to the patient?

Physicians not only have a responsibility to attempt to cure patients but, in the event a cure is not possible, to help in maximizing the quality of life of each patient. It is agreed by physicians dealing with dying patients that when a patient faces a terminal illness with little hope of long-term survival, it is important for the patient to know that his physician will assist him in order to live as fully as possible until the patient dies.

189. What has medicine learned from the study of AIDS?

Medicine includes illnesses both rare and common that are poorly understood and that have resulted in immense human suffering. Although AIDS is another entry to this long list, the study of AIDS may prove crucial in providing insights into the understanding and prevention of diseases as diverse as rheumatoid arthritis, multiple sclerosis, and systemic lupus erythematosus. All of these diseases are linked by a common thread, an immunological abnormality, and in many cases an infectious agent has been implicated but not isolated.

Immunity remains one of the most complex processes of the body. By understanding the immunological defect caused by the AIDS virus, fundamentally important discoveries applicable to all of medicine may occur and may provide revolutionary approaches to old diseases. The recognition that dementia can be the result of direct infection with the AIDS virus may also lead to better understanding and potential treatment for a number of neurological illnesses, including Alzheimer's disease.

AIDS is a disease that involves much more than purely medical issues. It already affects directly or indirectly millions of people worldwide. Few diseases have raised such important social and economic questions whose answers may change the way we now live.

We began our book with a prologue by Daniel Defoe, a quote from over two centuries ago describing a transmissible disease that ravaged Europe and became an infamous chapter in medical history. It seems fitting that we end our book on a more hopeful, and realistic, note that speaks optimistically to the efforts directed toward the eventual development of an AIDS vaccine and therapy:

Once the (AIDS) virus was isolated, tests . . . were developed with hectic speed to allow both assessment of the epidemic and development of control strategies. The interval from recognition of the first few cases of AIDS to the discovery of its cause was less than three years, and the second stage of advance to large-scale antibody testing was accomplished in less than a year. It is safe to assert that never in human history has science moved from recognition of a major medical problem to comprehensive understanding so swiftly. That the solution may not be at hand is testimony to the complexity of the problem, not an indictment of science.

June Osborn, MD
Issues in Science and Technology, Winter 1986

Perspectives

The acquired immunodeficiency syndrome was first formally recognized in 1981 when some persons were noticed to develop an unusual constellation of infections. The first few cases described were followed quickly by others so that by 1984, when the causative virus was linked to the disease, thousands of cases of the disease had been diagnosed. As more persons were identified with the disease and followed through time, the bleak prognosis for AIDS became apparent. A short time after the cause of the disease was discovered, numerous laboratories began devoting much effort to understand the nature of the AIDS virus and its singular destructiveness. Although scientists may take pride in the rapid isolation and virological characterization of the virus, patients with AIDS have the same prognosis now that they had when the virus was first found. Despite our optimism that scientific advances will occur, it still must be appreciated that there is currently no effective treatment to reverse the effects of the virus on the immune system. To have AIDS is to be guaranteed death in months to several years.

AIDS must now be considered to be of pandemic proportions. The initial appearance of the virus in well-defined risk groups, such as homosexual men and intravenous drug abusers in the United States, may have given the impression of some sort of special susceptibility of those groups to the disease, but that is clearly not the case. AIDS has occurred on all the inhabited continents and in people from all situations of life. Just as the AIDS virus has been shown to ignore all geographical boundaries, it has also been shown to have permeated any population that it enters when no precautions are taken to prevent its spread. As of early 1987, it had been estimated that at least 1.5 million people in the United States were infected and that Central Africa contained areas where nearly one quarter of the people were carrying the virus. Current estimates on the risk of developing AIDS during the course of infection with the virus indicate that large areas of Africa may well be significantly depopulated in the next decade. Not since the 1600s when a large fraction of the total population of Europe was decimated by the Black Plague has mankind faced a medical challenge of such significant proportions.

Even though scientists are at work and physicians are testing new compounds that could someday in the very indefinite future change the course of infection with the virus, people must not become complacent. Until a vaccine that has been rigorously tested and proven effective over several years exists, everyone must consider the possibility of becoming infected with the virus. They must understand how the virus is and is not transmitted, and they must learn about the deadly consequences of infection with HIV. They must learn that to be infected is to face a lifelong condition that exposes them and their most loved ones to possible death from the virus. They must know that the virus becomes an integral part of the body and that there is currently no way to rid the body of its presence.

In the absence of effective therapy, only one option is viable—education. Absolute priority must be given to getting the facts out. While AIDS is an incurable disease, it is also a preventable disease. Only a lack of care in considering the behavior between oneself and others once one is aware of the ways that the virus is transmitted will lead to infection of another person. Stopping the epidemic is a social concern of course, but in the final analysis society is composed of individuals who must collectively behave in a manner that will halt the spread of the virus. If not one more person were infected with the virus, AIDS would become extinct in this generation.

Glossary

acquired: not inherited but developed in the individual through some external influence

Acquired Immunodeficiency Syndrome (AIDS): an acquired syndrome of immunodeficiency resulting in susceptibility to severe infections and caused by a virus. This immunodeficiency is not related to the presence of other diseases or the use of medications that are known to depress immunity.

acute: having a rapid onset, a short course, and pronounced symptoms

acute (AIDS virus) infection: a transient illness characterized by nonspecific symptoms such as headache, skin rash, fever, malaise, enlarged lymph nodes, and diarrhea, and thought to represent an initial reaction to infection with the AIDS virus

AIDS-related complex (ARC): an acquired syndrome resembling AIDS but lacking the presence of an opportunistic infection or Kaposi's sarcoma. Persons with ARC often have chronic systemic symptoms such as lymph node enlargement, fever, diarrhea, lethargy, and localized infections less severe than seen in persons with AIDS.

Alzheimer's disease: a disease of middle-aged and elderly individuals characterized by progressive dementia and diffuse cerebral cortical atrophy, and microscopically by the presence of plaques, loss of neurons, and neurofibrillary tangles

antibody: a protein formed by lymphocytes that has the capacity to react against certain antigens present in bacteria, viruses, or other foreign substances. Antibodies are induced by exposure to specific chemicals unique to the invading microorganism or substance, and react specifically with these chemicals.

(AIDS) antibody positivity: the state in which an individual has been found to have antibodies, and thus prior exposure, to the AIDS virus

antigen: any substance that, when introduced into a foreign species, can elicit the formation of antibody specific for that substance

arthritis: a disease characterized by inflammation of the joints

artificial insemination: the injection of semen into the vagina or uterus to induce pregnancy by nonsexual means, usually through instrumentation

asymptomatic: having no symptoms of disease

azidothymidine (AZT): an experimental antiviral drug

B-lymphocyte: a cell type involved in immunity, and principally involved in the production of antibody (see *lymphocytes*)

benign: noncancerous, mild, gentle

bacteria: microscopic, one-celled organisms that are widely prevalent in nature, are members of the animal kingdom, and include many types able to cause disease in plants and animals

bisexual: having a sexual attraction to both males and females

Candida albicans: a fungus that is a part of the normal flora of the mucous membranes in the respiratory, gastrointestinal, and female genital tracts. In such locations it may gain dominance, producing pathological conditions and may be associated with severe systemic disease in immunosuppressed persons.

candidiasis: a condition produced by infection with Candida albicans, capable of involving a wide range of tissues of the body, including the skin, mucous membranes, nails, bronchi, lungs, heart, vagina, gastrointestinal tract, brain, and bloodstream

cardiopulmonary resuscitation: a prescribed sequence of steps designed to reestablish normal breathing in a person following cessation of either heart or lung function. It includes the establishment of an open airway, chest massage, and drug treatments.

carrier: an infected person who shows no signs or symptoms of disease but who harbors the infecting microorganism, and therefore is capable of spreading the disease

Centers for Disease Control: a federal agency located in Atlanta, Georgia, that plans, conducts, coordinates, and evaluates national programs for the prevention and control of transmissible diseases and other preventable conditions

cerebrospinal fluid: the fluid within the ventricles of the brain and between the arachnoid membrane and pia mater of the brain and spinal cord

chemotherapy: treatment of disease by any drug, colloquially used most often with reference to cancer chemotherapy

clotting factors: substances in the bloodstream that are important in the process of blood clotting and whose absence due to inherited or other disease produces prolonged bleeding

colonization: the presence of microorganisms in a host without resultant disease

compromised: lessened, as in an individual's decreased ability to fight infection resulting from compromised immunity

critical exposure: exposure of an individual to another infected person through known means of AIDS virus transmission, such as sexual intercourse or sharing of intravenous needles

cross-reactivity: a reaction between an antibody and an antigen that is closely related to, but not identical with, the specific antigen being tested for

cryoprecipitate: a substance derived from blood and rich in factor VIII, of importance for use in certain hemophiliacs

Cryptosporidium: a class of protozoa, containing several types capable of being opportunistic and producing severe inflammation of the small intestine and colon in compromised hosts

Cryptococcus neoformans: a fungus that may infect the skin, lungs, or bones, but which has a predilection for the central nervous system, causing primarily meningitis. In the severely immunocompromised host, it may disseminate via the bloodstream to any site in the body.

cytomegalovirus: a virus capable of being opportunistic and causing disseminated disease in immunocompromised hosts

dementia: an acquired progressive impairment of intellectual function with marked compromise in at least three of the following spheres of mental activity: language, memory, visuospatial skills, personality, and cognition (such as calculation and abstraction)

disorientation: the loss of normal relationship to one's surroundings, particularly the ability to comprehend time, place, and people

DNA: deoxyribonucleic acid, a type of chemical found in all plants, animals, bacteria, fungi, protozoa, and many viruses, able to reproduce in the presence of appropriate substrates, and carrying coded genetic information

ELISA: enzyme-linked immunosorbent assay, a test employed to detect the presence of AIDS virus antibody

empirical: based on observation

endemic: peculiar to a certain region; said of a disease that occurs constantly in any particular region

epidemic: a disease occurring or tending to occur in extensive outbreaks, or in an unusually high incidence at certain times and places

Epstein-Barr virus: a virus that is the cause of infectious mononucleosis and that has been suggested as capable of causing other diseases in immunocompromised hosts

factor VIII: a chemical important for blood clotting, present in the blood of normal persons, and deficient in the blood of patients with hemophilia A

factor IX: a chemical important for blood clotting, present in the blood of normal individuals, and deficient in the blood of patients with hemophilia B

fungi: one-celled organisms belonging to the plant kingdom, whose members contain a number of species capable of causing severe disease in immunocompromised hosts

gamma interferon: a type of protein formed by animal cells in the presence of a virus that limits viral reproduction and that is capable of inducing in noninfected cells of the same animal resistance to a variety of viruses

generalized lymphadenopathy syndrome: a syndrome of generalized lymphadenopathy (enlargement of lymph nodes) seen in increasing frequency in risk groups for AIDS, and thought to represent a condition related to infection with the AIDS virus

genetic: inherited characteristics of an individual

glaucoma: an eye disease, characterized by increased intraocular pressure and degeneration of the optic nerve head, which may result in defects in vision

gonorrhea: a sexually transmitted disease caused by the bacterium *Neisseria gonorrhea* and characterized by inflammation of the genital tract with possible secondary involvement of other tissues, including the heart, outer lining of the brain, and joints

helper T-lymphocyte: a subtype of lymphocytes active in the process of and stimulation of immunity; the cell principally infected and killed by the AIDS virus (see *lymphocytes*)

hemophilia: a hereditary bleeding disorder caused by factor VIII or factor IX deficiency and characterized clinically by bleeding into a variety of body sites

hepatitis B: a form of virally caused liver disease that can be contracted through sexual transmission and by the intravenous administration of human blood or blood products contaminated with the hepatitis B virus

herpes simplex virus: a virus causing a variety of human diseases notable for their persistence in a dormant state and tendency to recur at irregular intervals. Of the two main strains, type 1 usually causes infection of the mouth, skin, eye, and brain, while type 2 has an affinity for the genital tract. Both strains are capable of causing severe disease in immunocompromised hosts.

herpes zoster: an acute disease characterized by painful, vesicular eruptions on the skin or mucous membranes and caused by the varicella zoster virus.

heterosexual: having a sexual orientation toward the opposite sex

high risk: see *risk group*

histoplasmosis: an infection with the fungus *Histoplasma capsulatum,* capable of producing disease varying from a mild respiratory infection in most affected hosts to widespread disease of many organs, usually in immunocompromised hosts

HIV: Human Immunodeficiency Virus, the causative agent of AIDS, and synonymous with HTLV-III/LAV, LAV, and ARV

homosexual: having a sexual attraction toward the same sex

host: an organism on or in which another microorganism lives and from which the invading microorganism obtains nourishment during all or part of its existence

HPA-26: an antiviral drug currently under investigation for its effectiveness against AIDS

HTLV-III: Human Lymphotropic Virus-III, the causative agent of AIDS, named by the American research team who isolated it

immune system: a combination of cells and proteins that assist the host organism's ability to fight foreign substances, including microorganisms such as viruses and bacteria

immunity: the condition of a living organism whereby it resists and overcomes infection or disease

immunodeficiency: any deficiency of immune reaction, involving antibody-mediated or cell-mediated immunity only, or both, as in acquired immunodeficiency syndrome

immunoglobulin: any one of the proteins of animal origin having antibody activity that, when administered to an individual following exposure to a transmissible agent such as the virus causing hepatitis, may be capable of minimizing the risk of acquiring the diseases that the agent produces

incidence rate: the number of new cases of a disease that occur per population at risk, usually within a year and reported as the number of new cases per 100,000 population

incubation period: the period of time between infection and onset of symptoms

infection: the invasion of a host by organisms such as viruses, fungi, protozoa, or bacteria, with resultant disease

interferon: a protein, formed by animal cells in the presence of a virus, or other inducing agent, that prevents viral reproduction and is capable of protecting noninfected cells from viral infection. Several kinds of interferon exist (gamma, alpha, beta . . .)

interleukin-2: a substance produced by lymphocytes, that promotes long-term proliferation of T-lymphocytes with beneficial effects on immune functioning

intravenous: into a vein

intravenous drug abusers: individuals who inject substances into their bloodstream through a vein, typically with needles contaminated with blood from another intravenous drug abuser and capable of transmitting a variety of infectious diseases

in vitro: a process or reaction occurring in a glass, test tube, or petri dish rather than in the human body

isosporiasis: infection by any member of the group of protozoan *Isospora*

Isospora belli: a relatively rare species of the protozoan *Isospora,* capable of invading and causing disease of the small intestine and colon in man

Kaposi's sarcoma: a previously rare cancer primarily of the skin and lymph nodes that occurs frequently in those with

AIDS. This cancer often manifests itself clinically as pain-less purple to brown skin lesions and its presence is re-garded as evidence of AIDS even in the absence of an opportunistic infection.

LAV: Lymphadenopathy-Associated Virus, the name given the virus causing AIDS by its French discoverers. Lym-phadenopathy refers to the initial symptom of enlarged lymph nodes seen in many patients later diagnosed with AIDS.

lesbian: one who practices female homosexuality

lymph: a clear, transparent fluid collected from tissues throughout the body and flowing in special lymph vessels, eventually connecting and adding to the venous circulation

lymph node: masses of tissue intercalated in the course of vessels containing lymph. These nodes principally contain lymphocytes and are the masses through which lymph filters, permitting destruction of certain foreign agents by lymphatic cells.

lymphadenopathy: lymph node enlargement in response to any disease or foreign substance

lymphocyte: a type of white blood cell found in blood, lymph, and other specialized tissue such as bone marrow and ton-sils. Two major classes, B- and T-lymphocytes, are crucial components of the immune system. The B-lymphocytes are the cells primarily responsible for antibody production, while the T-lymphocytes cells are involved in the direct attack against invading organisms. A subtype of T-lym-phocyte, the helper T-lymphocyte, is the main cell infected and destroyed by the AIDS virus.

lymphoma: any tumor, usually malignant, of the lymphatic tissues

lymphotropism: the affinity of an invading organism for lym-phocytes

meningitis: any inflammation of the membranes lining the spinal cord and brain

molluscum contagiosum: a virally caused skin disease, whose affected sites principally include the face and anogenital area. The disease is sexually transmissible and usually asymptomatic except in immunocompromised hosts who may develop extensive involvement.

monogamy: the condition of having only one sexual partner

mortality: death rate

mucous membranes: the membranes lining those cavities and canals communicating with the air, such as the mouth and anus

multiple sclerosis: a demyelinating disease of unknown cause involving the central nervous system, most often of young adults, of varying severity and remissions, characterized clinically by episodes of focal disorder of the optic nerves, spinal cord, and brain, producing transient neurological symptoms such as dizziness, double vision, weakness or numbness

Mycobacterium avium-intracellulare: a species of Mycobacteria, a bacterial group, capable of causing severe lung disease in immunocompromised hosts

nanometer: one billionth of a meter

National Institutes of Health: a division of the United States Department of Health, Education, and Welfare, located in the Washington, DC area, that is devoted to both clinical and basic science research in public health and the diseases of man

non-Hodgkins lymphoma: a type of lymphoma

nucleic acid: a chemical compound found in all viruses, and plant and animal cells, of which RNA and DNA are the two princinal types

opportunistic: the quality of an organism such as a virus, bacterium, or fungus to produce disease when infecting an immunologically compromised host or when placed in a particular body location in large numbers. Such organisms generally do not produce disease when colonizing an immunologically normal host.

pandemic: epidemic over a wide geographic area, usually considered world-wide

placebo: a pharmacologically inactive substance, often used in studies to compare against clinical responses to the effects of pharmacologically active substances

placenta: the blood-filled organ that connects the fetus by the umbilical cord to the uterine wall, that is the source of mother-fetus blood exchange facilitating the transport of fetal nourishment from the mother

Pneumocystis carinii: a protozoan found widely in nature, causing no disease in normal individuals, but causing debilitating disease, usually of the lungs, in immunocompromised persons

pneumonia: a type of inflammation of the lungs, most often associated with infection by a microorganism

prenatal: existing or occurring before birth

prevalence rate: frequency of a disease in a population, usually expressed as the number of cases per 100,000 population

protein: one of a group of complex chemicals found in various forms in all living matter, including viruses. These chemicals form the principal components of all tissues.

prospective: looking and observing forward through time

protozoan: a one-celled organism of the animal kingdom containing many species widely distributed in nature, and ca pable of causing severe disease in immunocompromised hosts

quarantine: any limitation of movement or isolation imposed on an individual to keep a contagious disease from spreading

retrospective: looking back on the past

retrovirus: a class of viruses, containing RNA as its core nucleic acid. This class contains the causative agent of AIDS, and other viruses that cause immunodeficiency conditions in nonhuman animals

ribivirin: an experimental antiviral drug currently being tested for its effectiveness against AIDS

risk group: a group of individuals sharing a common feature that places them at an increased probability for acquiring a given disease compared to the general population

RNA: nucleic acid found in animal and plant cells, chemically different from DNA, but also important for the coding of genetic information

seropositivity: synonymous with antibody positivity

seronegativity: the absence of antibody positivity, synonymous with antibody negativity

serum: the cell-free fluid of the bloodstream, such as that appearing in a test tube after blood clots

Simian Acquired Immunodeficiency Syndrome: an immunodeficiency syndrome found in monkeys in which a retrovirus has been implicated as the causative agent

suramin: an antiviral agent currently being experimentally tested for its effectiveness against AIDS

syndrome: a group of symptoms and signs, which, when considered together, are known or presumed to characterize a disease

systemic lupus erythematosus: a disease of unknown cause characterized clinically by fever, muscle and joint pains, skin rashes, anemia, and leukopenia. The disease results in changes in connective tissue and primarily involves the kidneys, spleen, skin, and heart.

T-cell: a type of lymphocyte crucial to immunity and principally involved in the direct attack upon invading organisms (see *lymphocytes*)

thrush: a fungal infection due to *Candida albicans*, occurring most often in infants and characterized by small, whitish spots on the tongue and inner surface of the cheeks

Toxoplasma gondii: a protozoan widely found in nature, normally not disease-producing in healthy persons, but resulting in Toxoplasmosis, a devastating disease of the nervous system and eyes in immunocompromised hosts

tropism: having an affinity for some site

United States Public Health Service: the agency concerned with the development of a federal public health program and the handling of most health problems within the jurisdiction of the federal government

vaccine: a preparation administered to induce immunity against a particular agent; this agent may be a suspension of living or dead organisms or a solution of either pollens or viral or bacterial antigens. The administered materials are intended to induce immunity by antibody production without producing the disease against which the recipient is immunized.

varicella zoster virus: a virus that causes chicken pox and herpes zoster infections

venereal: pertaining to, or produced by, sexual intercourse *virus:* any of a vast group of minute structures composed of a protein coat encasing a core of DNA, RNA, or both, capable of infecting all animals and plants, including bacteria, totally dependent upon the cells of the infected host for their ability to reproduce, capable of causing devastating disease in immunocompromised individuals, and not affected by antibiotics

visna: a progressive disease of the brain and spinal cord of sheep, caused by a virus with a long incubation period. During this incubation period, when the animal is infected, it appears well without signs of disease

Western blot: a test designed to detect exposure to the AIDS virus by assessing the presence of AIDS virus antibody

References

Note: All references are keyed to the numbered questions.

1.

CDC. Pneumocystis pneumonia—Los Angeles. *Morbidity and Mortality Weekly Report* 30:250–252, 1981.

CDC. Kaposi's sarcoma and Pneumocystis pneumonia among homosexual men—New York and California. *Morbidity and Mortality Weekly Report* 25:305–308, 1981.

CDC. Results of a Gallup poll on acquired immunodeficiency syndrome—New York City, United States, 1985. *Morbidity and Mortality Weekly Report* 34:513–514, 1985.

AIDS ranked near cancer as nation's top health problem. *American Medical News,* October 18, 1985, p.2.

2.

Gallin, J. The compromised host. In Beeson, P., McDermott, W., Wyngaarden, J. (eds.). *Cecil Textbook of Medicine* (15th ed.). Philadelphia: W.B. Saunders, 1979, pp. 145–152.

3.

Tonegawa, S. The molecules of the immune system. *Scientific American* 253:October 1985, pp. 122–131.

Jaret, P. Our immune system: the wars within. *National Geographic,* June 1986, pp. 702–735.

4.

Gottlieb, M. (moderator). The acquired immunodeficiency syndrome. *Annals of Internal Medicine* 99:208–220, 1983

5.

Fauci, A.S. (moderator) NIH conference. Acquired immunodeficiency syndrome: epidemiologic, clinical, immunologic, and therapeutic considerations. *Annals of Internal Medicine* 100:92–106, 1984.

Gottlieb, M.S., Groopman, J.E., Weinstein, W.H., et al. The acquired immunodeficiency syndrome. *Annals of Internal Medicine* 99:208–220, 1984.

6.

Jaffe, H., Choi, K., Thomas, P., et al. National case-control study of Kaposi's sarcoma and pneumocystis carinii pneumonia in homosexual men: part 1, epidemiological results. *Annals of Internal Medicine* 99:145–158, 1983.

7.

Ibid.

Microbial diseases. In Beeson, P., McDermott, W., Wyngaarden, J. (eds.). *Cecil Textbook of Medicine* (15th ed.). Philadelphia: W.B. Saunders, 1979, pp. 227–638.

Benenson, A. (ed.). *Control of Communicable Diseases in Man.* (12th ed.). Washington, DC.: American Public Health Association, 1975.

8.

Fauci, A.S. (moderator). NIH conference. Acquired immunodeficiency syndrome: epidemiologic, clinical, immunologic, and therapeutic considerations. *Annals of Internal Medicine* 100:92–106, 1984.

9.

Joklik, W. (ed.). *Virology.* (2nd ed.). Norwalk, CT: Appleton-Century-Crofts, 1985.

10.

Ibid.

11.

Pictures of the AIDS virus taken with electron microscopy by Dr. Lennart Nilsson appear in: Jaret, P. Our immune system: the wars within. *National Geographic,* June 1986, pp. 702–735.

12.

Viral diseases. In Beeson, P., McDermott, W., Wyngaarden, J. (eds.). *Cecil Textbook of Medicine* (15th ed.). Philadelphia: W.B. Saunders, 1979, pp. 227–306.

Wong-Staal, F., Gallo, R. Human T-lymphotropic viruses. *Nature* 317:395–403, 1985.

Gallo, R., Wong-Staal, F. A. human T-lymphotropic retrovirus (HTLV-III) as the cause of the acquired immunodeficiency syndrome. *Annals of Internal Medicine* 103:679–689, 1985.

Barre-Sinoussi, F., Chermann, J-C., Rey, F., et al. Isolation of a T-lymphotropic retrovirus from a patient at risk for acquired immunodeficiency syndrome (AIDS). *Science* 220:868–871, 1983.

Gallo, R., Salahuddin, S., Popovic, M., et al. Frequent detection and isolation of cytopathic retroviruses (HTLV-III) from patients with AIDS and at risk for AIDS. *Science* 224:500–503, 1984.

Montagnier, L. Lymphadenopathy-associated virus: from molecular biology to pathogenicity. *Annals of Internal Medicine* 103:689–693, 1985.

Coffin, J., Haase, A., Levy, J., et al. Human immunodeficiency viruses (letter). *Science* 232:697, 1986.

14.

Levy, J., Hoffman, A., Kramer, S., et al. Isolation of lymphocytopathic retroviruses from San Francisco patients with AIDS. *Science* 225:840–842, 1984.

Kaminsky, L., McHugh, T., Stites, D., et al. High prevalence of antibodies to AIDS-associated retroviruses (ARV) in acquired immune deficiency syndrome and related conditions and not in other disease states. *Proceedings of the National Academy of Sciences USA* 82:5535–5539, 1985.

Weiss, S., Goedert, J., Sarngadharan, M., et al. Screening test for HTLV-III (AIDS agent) antibody: specificity, sensitivity, and applications. *Journal of the American Medical Association* 253:221–225, 1985.

Essex, M., McLane, M., Lee, T., et al. Antibodies to cell membrane antigens associated with human T-cell leukemia virus in patients with AIDS. *Science* 220:859–862, 1983.

15.

Tonegawa, S. The molecules of the immune system. *Scientific American* 253:October 1985, pp. 122–131.

16.

Laurence, J. The immune system in AIDS. *Scientific American* 253:84–93, 1985.

Bowen, D., Lane, H., Fauci, A. Immunopathogenesis of the acquired immunodeficiency syndrome. *Annals of Internal Medicine* 103:704–709, 1985.

Kalish, R., Schlossman, S. The T₄ lymphocyte in AIDS. *The New England Journal of Medicine* 313:112–113, 1985.

Kornfield, H., Van de Stouwe, R., Lange, M., et al. T-lymphocyte sub-populations in homosexual men. *The New England Journal of Medicine* 307:729–731, 1982.

Weiss, A., Hollander, A., Stobo, J. Acquired immunodeficiency syndrome: epidemiology, virology, and immunology. *Annual Review of Medicine* 36:545–562, 1985.

17.

Bowen, D., Lane, H., Fauci, A. Immunopathogenesis of the acquired immunodeficiency syndrome. *Annals of Internal Medicine* 103:704–709, 1985.

Murray, H., Rubin, B., Masur, H., et al. Impaired production of lymphokines and immune (gamma) interferon in the acquired immunodeficiency syndrome. *The New England Journal of Medicine* 310:883-889, 1984.

Lane, H., Masur, H., Edgar, L., et al. Abnormalities of B-cell activation and immunoregulation in patients with the acquired immunodeficiency syndrome. *The New England Journal of Medicine* 309:453–458, 1983.

Mitsuyasa, R., Volberding, P., Groopman, J., et al. Bone marrow transplantation from identical twins in the treatment of the acquired immunodeficiency syndrome and Kaposi's sarcoma. *Journal of Cell biochemistry (suppl.)* 8A:19, 1984.

Lane, H., Fauci, A. Immunologic reconstitution in the acquired immunodeficiency syndrome. *Annals of Internal Medicine* 103:714–718, 1985.

Immune stimulators. *FDA Bulletin* 15:31–32, 1985.

18.

Hirsch, M., Kaplan, J. Prospects of therapy for infection with human T-lymphotropic virus type III. *Annals of Internal Medicine* 103:750–755, 1985.

Microbial diseases. In Beeson, P., McDermott, W., Wyngaarden, J., (eds.). *Cecil Textbook of Medicine* (15th ed.). Philadelphia: W.B. Saunders, 1979, pp. 227–638.

19.

For a description of vaccine development see: Godsen G. Molecular approaches to malaria vaccines. *Scientific American* 252(5):52–59, 1985.

Laurence, J. The immune system in AIDS. *Scientific American* 253:84–93, 1985.

Joklik, W. Antiviral chemotherapy, interferon, and vaccines. In Joklik, W. (ed.). *Virology.* (2nd ed.). Norwalk, CT: Appleton-Century-Crofts, 1985, pp. 117–119.

20.

Francis, D., Petricciani, J. The prospects for and pathways toward a vaccine for AIDS. *The New England Journal of Medicine* 315:1586–1590, 1985.

Beardsley, T. AIDS progress. Synthetic vaccine only a distant prospect. *Nature* 314:659, 1985.

Benn, S., Rutledge, R., Folks, T., et al. Genomic heterogeneity of AIDS retroviral isolates from North America and Zaire. *Science* 230:949–951, 1985.

Wong-Staal, F., Gallo, R. Human T-lymphotropic viruses. *Nature* 317:395–403, 1985.

Hahn, B., Shaw, G., Taylor, M., et al. Genetic variation in HTLV-III/LAV over time in patients with AIDS or at risk for AIDS. *Science* 232:1548–1553, 1986.

21.

Gottlieb, M. (moderator). The acquired immunodeficiency syndrome. *Annals of Internal Medicine* 99:208–220, 1983.

Goedert, J., Blattner, W. The epidemiology of the acquired immunodeficiency syndrome. In DeVita, V., Hellman, S., Rosenberg, S. (eds.). *AIDS: Etiology, Diagnosis, Treat-*

ment, and Prevention. Philadelphia: J.B. Lipponcott Co., pp. 1–30, 1985.

22.
Letvin, N., Eaton, K., Aldrich, W., et al. Acquired immunodeficiency syndrome in a colony of macaque monkeys. *Proceedings of the National Academy of Sciences* 80:2118–2722, 1983.

Letvin, N., Daniel, M., Sehgal, P., et al. Induction of AIDS-like disease in macaque monkeys with T-cell tropic retrovirus STLV-III. *Science* 230:71–73, 1985.

Kanki, P., Alroy, J., Essex, M. Isolation of T-lymphotropic retrovirus related to HTLV-III/LAV from wild-caught African green monkeys. *Science* 230:951–954, 1985.

Marx, P., Maul, D., Osborn, K., et al. Simian AIDS: isolation of a type D retrovirus and transmission of the disease. *Science* 223:1083–1086, 1984.

23.
Joklik, W. (ed.). *Virology.* (2nd ed.). Norwalk, CT: Appleton-Century-Crofts, 1985.

24.
Barry, D. Influenza viruses. Joklik, W. (ed.). *Virology,* (2nd ed.). Norwalk, CT: Appleton-Century-Crofts, 1985, p. 243.

25.
Kanki, P., Alroy, J., Essex, M. Isolation of T-lymphotropic retrovirus related to HTLV-III/LAV from wild-caught African green monkeys. *Science* 230:951–954, 1985.

Clumeck, N., Sonnet, J., Taelman, H., et al. Acquired immunodeficiency syndrome in African patients. *The New England Journal of Medicine* 310:492–497, 1984.

Biggar, R. The AIDS problem in Africa. *Lancet* 1:79–82, 1986.

26.
Fauci, A. (moderator). NIH conference. The acquired immunodeficiency syndrome: an update. *Annals of Internal Medicine* 102:800–813, 1985.

27.
Ibid.

28.
Ibid.

29.
Reichert, C., O'Leary, T., Levens, D., et al. Autopsy pathology in the acquired immune deficiency syndrome. *American Journal of Pathology* 112:357–382, 1983.

Koretz, S. Treatment of serious cytomegalovirus infections with 9-(1,3 dihydroxy-2-propxymethyl) guanine in patients with AIDS and other immunodeficiencies. *The New England Journal of Medicine* 314:801–805, 1986.

Kovacs, J. *Pneumocystis carinii* pneumonia: a comparison between patients with the acquired immunodeficiency syndrome and patients with other immunodeficiencies. *Annals of Internal Medicine* 100:663–671, 1984.

30.
Diagnosing the infections of AIDS. *Cancer Reporter* 1(1):4–5, 1985.

Kaplan, L., Wofsy, C., Volberding, P. Treatment of patients with the acquired immunodeficiency syndrome and associated manifestations. *Journal of the American Medical Association* 257:1367–1374, 1987.

DeHovitz, J., Pape, J., Boncy, M., et al. Clinical manifestations and therapy of *Isospora Belli* infection in patients with the acquired immunodeficiency syndrome. *The New England Journal of Medicine* 315(2):87–90, 1986.

31.
Quinn, T. Early symptoms and signs of AIDS and the AIDS-related complex. In Ebbersen, P., Biggar, R., Melbye, M. (eds.). *AIDS*. Copenhagen: Munksgaard, pp. 69–81, 1984.

Kotler, D., Gaetz, H., Lange, M., et al. Enteropathy associated with the acquired immunodeficiency syndrome. *Annals of Internal Medicine* 100:693–696, 1984.

Kovacs, J., Kovacs, A., Polis, M., et al. Cryptococcus in the acquired immunodeficiency syndrome. *Annals of Internal Medicine* 103:533–538, 1985.

Patterson, R. Neurological surgery. *Journal of the American Medical Association* 254:2310–2311, 1985.

Klein, R., Harris, C., Small, C., et al. Oral candidiasis in high-risk patients as the initial manifestation of the acquired immunodeficiency syndrome. *The New England Journal of Medicine* 311:354–358, 1984.

Ostrow, J., Vanagunas, A. Gastroenterology and hepatology. *Journal of the American Medical Association* 254(16): 2267–2269, 1985.

CDC. Oral viral lesion (hairy leukoplakia) associated with acquired immunodeficiency syndrome. *Morbidity and Mortality Weekly Report* 34(36):549–550, 1985.

Levy, R., Bredesen, D., Rosenblum, M. Neurological manifestations of the acquired immunodeficiency syndrome (AIDS): experience at UCSF and review of the literature. *Journal of Neurosurgery* 62:475–495, 1985.

Elkin, C., Leon, E., Grenell, S., et al. Intracranial lesions in the acquired immunodeficiency syndrome. Radiological (computed tomographic) features. *Journal of the American Medical Association* 253:393–396, 1985.

Navia, B., Petito, C., Gold, J., et al. Cerebral toxoplasmosis complicating the acquired immune deficiency syndrome: clinical and neuropathological findings in 27 patients. *Annals of Neurology* 19:224–238, 1986.

Nath, A., Jakovic, J., Pettigrew, L. Movement disorders and AIDS. *Neurology* 37:37–41, 1987.

32.

Welch, K., Finkbeiner, W., Alpers, C., et al. Autopsy findings in the acquired immune deficiency syndrome. *Journal of the American Medical Association* 252:1152–1159, 1984.

Murray, J., Felton, C., Garay, S., et al. Pulmonary complications of the acquired immunodeficiency syndrome: report of a National Heart, Lung, and Blood Institute Workshop. *The New England Journal of Medicine* 310:1682–1688, 1984.

Haverkos, H. Assessment of therapy for *Pneumocystis carinii* pneumonia. POP therapy project group. *The American Journal of Medicine* 78:501–508, 1984.

Shelhammer, J., Oghibene, F., Macher, A., et al. Persistence of *Pneumocystis carinii* in lung tissue of acquired immunodeficiency patients treated for pneumocystis pneumonia. *American Review of Respiratory Disease* 130:1161–1165, 1984.

Leads from the MMWR. CDC. Update: acquired immunodeficiency syndrome—United States. *Journal of the American Medical Association* 255:593–598, 1986.

33.
Diagnosing the infections of AIDS. *Cancer Reporter* 1(1):4–5, 1985.

34.
Price, R., Navia, B., Cho, E-S. AIDS encephalopathy. In Booss, J., Thornton, G (eds.). Infectious Diseases of the Central Nervous System. *Neurologic Clinics* 4(1):285–301, 1986.

Shaw, G., Harper, M., Hahn, B., et al. HTLV-III infection in brains of children and adults with AIDS encephalopathy. *Science* 227:177–181, 1985.

Levy, J., Hollander, H., Kaminsky, L., et al. Isolation of AIDS-associated retroviruses from cerebrospinal fluid and brain of patients with neurological symptoms. *Lancet* 2:586–588, 1985.

Ho, D., Rota, T., Schooley, R., et al. Isolation of HTLV-III from cerebrospinal fluid and neural tissues of patients with neurologic syndromes related to the acquired immunodeficiency syndrome. *The New England Journal of Medicine* 313:1492–1497, 1985.

Gajdusek, D., Amyx, H., Gibbs, C., et al. Infection of chimpanzees by human T-lymphotropic retroviruses in brain and other tissues from AIDS patients. *Lancet* 1:55-56, 1985.

Petito, C., Navia, B., Cho, E., et al. Vacuolar myelopathy pathologically resembling subacute combined degeneration in patients with the acquired immunodeficiency syndrome.

The New England Journal of Medicine 312:874–879, 1985.

Price, R., Navia, B. The acquired immunodeficiency syndrome dementia complex as the presenting or sole manifestation of human immunodeficiency virus infection. *Archives of Neurology* 44:65–69, 1987.

Eidelberg, D., Sotrel, A., Vogel, H., et al. Progressive polyradiculopathy in acquired immune deficiency syndrome. *Neurology* 36:912–916, 1986.

Navia, B., Jordan, B., Price, R. The AIDS dementia complex: I. Clinical features. *Annals of Neurology* 19:517–524, 1986.

Navia, B., Cho, E-S, Petito, C., et al. The AIDS complex. II. Neuropathology. *Annals of Neurology* 19:525–535, 1986.

35.

Resnick, L., DiMarzo–Veronese, F., Schupbach, J., et al. Intra-blood–brain–barrier synthesis of HTLV-III-specific IgG in patients with neurological symptoms associated with AIDS or AIDS-related complex. *The New England Journal of Medicine* 313:1498–1505, 1985.

Gonda, M., Wong-Staal, F., Gallo, R., et al. Sequence homology and morphologic similarity of HTLV-III and visna virus, a pathogenic lentivirus. *Science* 227:173–177, 1985.

Stephens, R., Casey, J., Rice, N. Equine infectious anemia virus *gag* and *pol* genes: relatedness to visna and AIDS virus. *Science* 231:589–594, 1986.

Koenig, S., Gendelman, H., Orenstein, J., et al. Detection of AIDS virus in the macrophages in brain tissue from AIDS patients with encephalopathy. *Science* 233:1089–1093, 1986.

36.

Leads from the MMWR. CDC. Update: acquired immunodeficiency syndrome—United States. *Journal of the American Medical Association* 255:593–598, 1986.

Groopman, J., Gottlieb, M., Goodman, J., et al. Recombinant alpha-2 interferon therapy for Kaposi's sarcoma associated with the acquired immunodeficiency syndrome. *Annals of Internal Medicine* 100:671–676, 1984.

Stahl, R., Friedman-Kien, A., Dubin, R., et al. Immunologic abnormalities in homosexual men. Relationship to Kaposi's sarcoma. *The American Journal of Medicine* 73:171–178, 1985.

Nitrate aerosol use linked to Kaposi's in AIDS patients. *Internal Medicine News* 19:61, 1986.

Krown, S., Real, F., Cunningham-Rundles, S., et al. Preliminary observations on the effect of recombinant leukocyte A interferon in homosexual men with Kaposi's sarcoma. *The New England Journal of Medicine* 308:1071–1076, 1985.

Volberding, P., Abrams, D., Conant, M., et al. Vinblastine therapy for Kaposi's sarcoma in the acquired immunodeficiency syndrome. *Annals of Internal Medicine* 103:335–338, 1985.

37.
Centers for Disease Control, Atlanta, Georgia, personal communication.

38.
Rivin, B., Monroe, J., Hubschman, B., et al. AIDS outcome: a first follow-up. *The New England Journal of Medicine* 311:857, 1984.

Safai, B., Johnson, K., Myskowski, P., et al. The natural history of Kaposi's sarcoma in the acquired immunodeficiency syndrome. *Annals of Internal Medicine* 103:744–750, 1985.

39.
Rivin, B., Monroe, J., Hubschman, B., et al. AIDS outcome: a first follow-up. *The New England Journal of Medicine* 311:857, 1984.

Osborn, J. The AIDS epidemic: an overview of the science. *Issues in Science and Technology* 40–55, Winter 1986.

40.
CDC. Revision of the case definition of acquired immunodeficiency syndrome for national reporting—United States *Morbidity and Mortality Weekly Report* 34:373–375, 1985

41.

Fauci, A. (moderator). NIH conference. Acquired immunodeficiency syndrome: an update. *Annals of Internal Medicine* 102:800–813, 1985.

Allen, J., Curran, J. Epidemiology of the acquired immunodeficiency syndrome (AIDS). In Gallin, J., Fauci, A. (eds.). *Acquired Immunodeficiency Syndrome.* New York: Raven Press, pp. 1–27, 1985. *(Advances in Host Defense Mechanisms,* vol. 5).

42.

Ibid.

43.

Murray, H., Hillman, J., Rubin, B., et al. Patients at risk for AIDS-related opportunistic infections. *The New England Journal of Medicine* 313:1504–1510, 1985.

44.

Allen, J., Curran, J. Epidemiology of the acquired immunodeficiency syndrome (AIDS). In Gallin, J., Fauci, A. (eds.). *Advances in Host Defense Mechanisms.* New York: Raven Press, pp. 1–27, 1985.

Metroka, C., Cunningham-Rundles, S., Pollack, M., et al. Generalized lymphadenopathy in homosexual men. *Annals of Internal Medicine* 99:585–91, 1983.

Gold, J., Weikel, C., Godbold, J., et al. Unexplained persistent lymphadenopathy in homosexual men and the acquired immune deficiency syndrome. *Medicine* 64:203–213, 1985.

5.

Schupbach, J., Haller, O., Vogt, M., et al. Antibodies to HTLV-III in Swiss patients with AIDS and pre-AIDS and in groups at risk for AIDS. *The New England Journal of Medicine* 312:265–270, 1985.

Metroka, C., Cunningham-Rundles, S., Pollack, M., et al. Generalized lymphadenopathy in homosexual men. *Annals of Internal Medicine* 99:585–91, 1983.

Abrams, D. Lymphadenopathy syndrome in male homosexuals. In Gallin, J., Fauci, A., (eds.). *Acquired Immunode-*

ficiency Syndrome. New York: Raven Press, pp. 75–97, 1985. *(Advances in Host Defense Mechanisms,* vol. 5).

Barre-Sinoussi, F., Chermann, J-C, Rey, F., et al. Isolation of a T-lymphotropic retrovirus from a patient at risk for acquired immune deficiency syndrome (AIDS). *Science* 220:868–871, 1983.

46.
Curran, J. The epidemiology and prevention of the acquired immunodeficiency syndrome. *Annals of Internal Medicine* 103:657–662, 1985.

Ho, D., Schooley, R., Rota, T., et al. HTLV-III in the semen and blood of a healthy homosexual man. *Science* 226:451–453, 1984.

Salahuddin, S., Groopman, J., Markham, P., et al. HTLV-III in symptom-free seronegative persons. *Lancet* 2:1418–1420, 1984.

Valle, S., Saxinger, C., Ranki, A., et al. Diversity of clinical spectrum of HTLV-III spectrum. *Lancet* 1:301–304, 1985.

Sivak, S., Wormser, G. How common is HTLV-III infection in the United States? *The New England Journal of Medicine* 313:1352, 1985.

47.
Ho, D., Sarngadharan, N., Resnick, L., et al. Primary human T-lymphotropic virus type III infection. *Annals of Internal Medicine* 103:880–883, 1985.

Carne, C., Tedder, R., Smith, A., et al. Acute encephalopathy coincident with seroconversion for anti-HTLV-III *Lancet* 2:1206–1208, 1985.

Cooper, D., Gold, J., MacLean, P., et al. Acute AIDS retrovirus infection: definition of a clinical illness associated with seroconversion. *Lancet* 1:537–540, 1985.

Tucker, J., Ludlam, C., Craig, A., et al. HTLV-III infection associated with glandular-fever-like illness in a haemophiliac. *Lancet* 1:585, 1985.

Lindskov, R., Lindhardt, B., Weismann, K., et al. Acute HTLV-III infection with roseola-like rash. *Lancet* 1:447 1986.

48.

CDC. Update: acquired immunodeficiency syndrome in the San Francisco Cohort study, 1978–1985. *Morbidity and Mortality Weekly Report* 34:573–575, 1985.

Jaffe, H., Darrow, W., Echenberg, D., et al. The acquired immunodeficiency syndrome in a cohort of homosexual men. A six-year follow-up study. *Annals of Internal Medicine* 103:719–722, 1985.

Goedert, J., Biggar, R., Weiss, S., et al. Three-year incidence of AIDS in five cohorts of HTLV-III-infected risk group members. *Science* 231:992–995, 1986.

Francis, D., Jaffe, H., Fultz, P., et al. The natural history of infection with the lymphadenopathy-associated virus human T-lymphotropic virus type III. *Annals of Internal Medicine* 103:719–722, 1985.

Weber, J., Rogers, L., Scott, K., et al. Three-year prospective study of HTLV-III/LAV infection in homosexual men. *Lancet* 1:1179–1182, 1986.

49.

Fincher, R., deSilva, M., Lobel, S., et al. AIDS-related complex in a heterosexual man seven weeks after a transfusion. *The New England Journal of Medicine* 313:1226, 1985.

Curran, J. The epidemiology and prevention of the acquired immunodeficiency syndrome. *Annals of Internal Medicine* 103:657–662, 1985.

50.

CDC. Classification system for human T-lymphotropic virus type III/lymphadenopathy-associated virus infections. *Morbidity and Mortality Weekly Report* 35(20):334–339, 1986.

51.

Centers for Disease Control, Atlanta, Georgia.

52.

Auerbach, D., Darrow, W., Jaffe, H., et al. Cluster of cases of the acquired immunodeficiency syndrome. Patients linked by sexual contact. *The American Journal of Medicine* 78:487–492, 1984.

53.

Goedert, J., Sarngadharan, M., Biggar, R., et al. Determinants of retrovirus (HTLV-III) antibody and immunodeficiency conditions in homosexual men. *Lancet* 2:711–716, 1984.

Jaffe, H., Choi, K., Thomas, P., et al. National case-control study of Kaposi's sarcoma and Pneumocystis carinii pneumonia in homosexual men: part I, epidemiological results. *Annals of Internal Medicine* 99:145–151, 1983.

54.

Ibid.

55.

CDC. Provisional Public Health Service inter-agency recommendations for screening donated blood and plasma for antibody to the virus causing acquired immunodeficiency syndrome. *Morbidity and Mortality Weekly Report* 34:1–4, 1985.

56.

Goedert, J., Sarnagadharan, M., Biggar, R., et al. Determinants of retrovirus (HTLV-III) antibody and immunodeficiency conditions in homosexual men. *Lancet* 2:711–716, 1984.

57.

Curran, J. The epidemiology and prevention of the acquired immunodeficiency syndrome. *Annals of Internal Medicine* 103:657–662, 1985.

58.

Harris, C., Butkus-Small, C., Klein, R., et al. Immunodeficiency in female sexual partners of men with the acquired immunodeficiency syndrome. *The New England Journal of Medicine* 308:1181–1184, 1983.

Curran, J. The epidemiology and prevention of the acquired immunodeficiency syndrome. *Annals of Internal Medicine* 103:657–662, 1985.

Pirot, P., Taelman, H., Minlangu, K., et al. Acquired immunodeficiency syndrome in heterosexual population in Zaire. *Lancet* 2:65–69, 1984.

59.
CDC. Leads from the MMWR. Acquired immunodeficiency syndrome in correctional facilities: a report of the National Institute of Justice and the American Correctional Association. *Journal of the American Medical Association* 255:2412–2419, 1986.

60.
Redfield, A., Markham, P., Salahuddin, S., et al. Heterosexually acquired HTLV-III/LAV disease (AIDS-related complex and AIDS): epidemiological evidence for female-to-male transmission. *Journal of the American Medical Association* 254:2094–2096, 1985.

Luzi, G., Ensoli, B., Turbessi, G., et al. Transmission of HTLV-III infection by heterosexual contact. *Lancet* 2:1018, 1985.

CDC. Heterosexual transmission of human T-lymphotropic virus type III/lymphadenopathy-associated virus. *Morbidity and Mortality Weekly Report* 34:561–563, 1985.

Clumeck, N., Van De Perre, P., Carael, M., et al. Heterosexual promiscuity among African patients with AIDS. *Lancet* 2:182, 1985.

Van De Perre, P., Clumeck, N., Carael, M., et al. Female prostitutes: a risk group for infection with HTLV-III. *Lancet* 2:524–527, 1985.

Calabrese, L., Gopalakrishna, K. Transmission of HTLV-III infection from man to woman to man. *The New England Journal of Medicine* 314:987, 1986.

Vogt, M., Witt, D., Craven, D., et al. Isolation of HTLV-III/LAV from cervical secretions of women at risk for AIDS. *Lancet* 1:525–527, 1986.

Wofsy, C., Cohen, J., Hauer, L., et al. Isolation of AIDS-associated retrovirus from genital secretions of women with antibodies to the virus. *Lancet* 1:527–529, 1986.

Gill, P., Levine, A., Meyer, P., et al. Human T-cell lymphotropic virus type-III associated disorders. *Archives of Internal Medicine* 146:1501–1504, 1986.

61.

Ginzburg, H., Weiss, S., MacDonald, M., et al. HTLV-III exposure among drug users. *Cancer Research* (in press). Cited in Landesman, S., Ginzburg, H., Weiss, S. The AIDS epidemic. *The New England Journal of Medicine* 312:521–524, 1985.

Van De Perre, P., Clumeck, N., Carael, M., et al. Female prostitutes: a risk group for infection with HTLV-III. *Lancet* 2:524-527, 1985.

Papaevangelou, G., Roumeliotou-Karayannis, A., Kallinikos, G., et al. LAV/HTLV-III infection in female prostitutes. *Lancet* 2:1018–1019, 1985.

Kreiss, J., Koech, D., Plummer, F., et al. AIDS virus infection in Nairobi prostitutes. *The New England Journal of Medicine* 314:414–418, 1986.

62.

Centers for Disease Control, Atlanta, Georgia.

63.

Melbye, M., Biggar, R., Ebbersen, P., et al. Seroepidemiology of HTLV-III antibody in Danish homosexual men: prevalence, transmission, and disease outcome. *British Medical Journal (Clinical Research)* 289:573–575, 1984.

Glauser, M., Francioli, P. Clinical and epidemiological survey of acquired immune deficiency syndrome in Europe. *European Journal of Clinical Microbiology* 3:55–58, 1984.

Biggar, R., Melbye, M., Ebbesen, P., et al. Low T-lymphocyte ratios in homosexual men: epidemiologic evidence for a transmissible agent. *Journal of the American Medical Association* 231:1441–1446, 1984.

64.

Redfield, R., Markham, P., Salahuddin, S., et al. Frequent transmission of HTLV-III among spouses of patients with AIDS-related complex (ARC) and the acquired immune deficiency syndrome: a family study. *Journal of the American Medical Association* 253:1571–1573, 1985.

Harris, C., Small, C., Klein, R., et al. Immunodeficiency in female sexual partners of men with the acquired immunodeficiency syndrome. *The New England Journal of Medicine* 308:1181–1184, 1983.

Redfield, R., Markham, P., Salahuddin, S., et al. Heterosexually acquired HTLV-III/LAV disease (AIDS-related complex and AIDS): Epidemiologic evidence for female-to-male transmission. *Journal of the American Medical Association* 254:2094–2096, 1985.

65.
Greene, J., Sidhu, G., Lewin, S. Mycobacterium avium-intracellulare: a cause of disseminated life-threatening infection in homosexuals and drug abusers. *Annals of Internal Medicine* 97:539–546, 1982.

Small, C., Klein, R., Friedland, G., et al. Community acquired opportunistic infections and defective cellular immunity in heterosexual drug abusers and homosexual men. *The American Journal of Medicine* 74:453–454, 1983.

66.
Friedland, G., Harris, C., Butkus-Small, C., et al. Intravenous drug abusers and the acquired immunodeficiency syndrome (AIDS). Demographic, drug use, and needle sharing patterns. *Archives of Internal Medicine* 145:1413–1417, 1985.

Mulleady, G., Green, J. Syringe sharing among London drug abusers. *Lancet* 2:1425, 1985.

67.
Ammann, A. The acquired immunodeficiency syndrome in infants and children. *Annals of Internal Medicine* 103:734–737, 1985.

Rogers, M. AIDS in children: a review of the clinical, epidemiologic, and public health aspects. *Pediatric Infectious Disease* 4:230–236, 1985.

Cowan, M., Hellmann, D., Chudwin, D., et al. Maternal transmission of acquired immune deficiency syndrome. *Pediatrics* 73:382–386, 1984.

Lapointe, N., Michand, J., Pelcovic, D., et al. Transplacental transmission of HTLV-III virus. *The New England Journal of Medicine* 312:1325–1326, 1985.

Jovaisas, E., Koch, M., Schafer, A., et al. LAV/HTLV-III in 20-week fetus. *Lancet* 2:1129, 1985.

CDC. Recommendations for assisting in the prevention of perinatal transmission of human T-lymphotropic virus type III/lymphadenopathy-associated virus and acquired immunodeficiency syndrome. *Morbidity and Mortality Weekly Report* 34:721–731, 1985.

Pahwa, S., Kaplan, M., Fikrig, S., et al. Spectrum of human T-cell lymphotropic virus type III infection in children: recognition of symptomatic, asymptomatic, and sero-negative parents. *Journal of the American Medical Association* 255:2229–2305, 1986.

68.
Marion, R., Wiznia, A., Hutcheon, G., et al. Human T-cell lymphotropic virus type III (HTLV-III) embryopathy: a new dysmorphic syndrome associated with intrauterine HTLV-III infection. *American Journal of Diseases in Children* 140:638–640, 1986.

69.
Fazakerly, J., Webb, H. Isolation of AIDS virus from cell-free breast milk of three healthy virus carriers. *Lancet* 2:891–892, 1985.

70.
CDC. Immunization Advisory Practices Committee. Immunization of children infected with human T-lymphotropic virus type III/lymphadenopathy-associated virus. *Annals of Internal Medicine* 106:75–78, 1987.

71.
CDC. Acquired immunodeficiency syndrome: meeting of the WHO collaborating centres on AIDS. *Morbidity and Mortality Weekly Report* 678, 1985.

CDC. Education and foster care of children infected with human T-lymphotropic virus type III/lymphadenopathy-associated virus. *Morbidity and Mortality Weekly Report* 34:517–521, 1985.

72.
CDC. Provisional Public Health Service inter-agency recommendations for screening donated blood and plasma for anti

body to the virus causing acquired imunodeficiency syndrome. *Morbidity and Mortality Weekly Report* 34:1–4, 1985.

Fischl, M., Dickenson, G., Scott, G., et al. Evaluation of heterosexual partners, children, and household contacts of adults with AIDS. *Journal of the American Medical Association* 257:640–644, 1987.

Friedland, G., Saltzman, B., Rogers, M., et al. Lack of transmission of HTLV-III/LAV infection to household contacts of patients with AIDS or AIDS-related complex with oral candidiasis. *The New England Journal of Medicine* 314:344–349, 1986.

CDC. Education and foster care of children infected with human T-lymphotropic virus type III/lymphadenopathy-associated virus. *Morbidity and Mortality Weekly Report* 34:517–521, 1985.

CDC. Recommendations for preventing transmission of infection with human T-lymphotropic virus type III/ lymphadenopathy-associated virus in the workplace. *Morbidity and Mortality Weekly Report* 34:682–695, 1985.

73.

Barre-Sinoussi, F., Nugeyre, M., Chermann, J. Resistance of AIDS virus at room temperature. *Lancet* 2:721–722, 1985.

Resnick, L., Veren, K., Salahuddin, S., et al. Stability and inactivation of HTLV-III/LAV under clinical and laboratory environments. *Journal of the American Medical Association* 255:1887–1891, 1986.

Ho, D., Byington, R., Schooley, R., et al. Infrequency of isolation of HTLV-III virus from saliva in AIDS. *The New England Journal of Medicine* 313:1606, 1985.

74.

Lifson, A., Castro, K., White, C., et al. 'No identified risk' AIDS cases. In *Program and abstracts of the 26th Interscience conference on Antimicrobial Agents and Chemotherapy*. September 28–October 1, 1986, p. 283.

75.

Hougie, C. Hemophilia and related conditions—congenital deficiencies of prothrombin (factor II), factor V, and factors VII to XII. In Williams, W., Beutler, E., Erslev, A., et al. (eds.). *Hematology*. (3rd ed.). New York: McGraw Hill, pp. 1381–1388, 1983.

76.

Curran, J., Evatt, B., Lawrence, D. Acquired immune deficiency syndrome: the past as prologue. *Annals of Internal Medicine* 98:401–402, 1983.

Ludlam, C., Steel, C., Cheingsong-Popov, R., et al. Human T-lymphotropic virus type III (HTLV-III) infection in seronegative hemophiliacs after transfusion of factor VIII. *Lancet* 2:233–236, 1985.

DeShazo, A., Andes, W., Norderg, J. An immunological evaluation of hemophiliac patients and their wives. Relationship to the acquired immunodeficiency syndrome. *Annals of Internal Medicine* 99:159–163, 1983.

Evatt, B., Ramsey, R., Lawrence, D., et al. The acquired immunodeficiency syndrome in patients with hemophilia. *Annals of Internal Medicine* 100:499–504, 1984.

Ragni, M., Lewis, J., Spero, J., et al. Decreased helper/suppressor cell ratios after treatment with factor VIII and IX concentrates and fresh frozen plasma. *The American Journal of Medicine* 76:206–210, 1984.

Lederman, M., Ratnoff, O., Evatt, B., et al. Acquisition of antibody to lymphadenopathy-associated virus in patients with classic hemophilia (factor VIII deficiency). *Annals of Internal Medicine* 102:753–757, 1985.

77–78.

Hougie, C. Hemophilia and related conditions—congenital deficiencies of prothrombin (factor II), factor V, and factors VII to XII. In Williams, W., Beutler, E., Erslev, A., et al. (eds.). *Hematology* (3rd ed.). New York: McGraw Hill pp. 1381–1388, 1983.

McGrady, G., Gjerset, G., Kennedy, S. Risk of exposure to HTLV-III/LAV and type of clotting factor used in hemophilia. *International Conference on AIDS*. Atlanta, Georgia, April 16, 1985.

Koerper, M., Kaminsky, L., Levy, J. Differential prevalence of antibody to AIDS-associated retrovirus in hemophiliac treated with factor VIII concentrate versus cryoprecipitate: recovery of infectious virus. *Lancet* 1:275, 1985.

Jason, J., McDougal, J., Holman, R., et al. Human T-lymphotropic retrovirus type III/lymphadenopathy associated virus antibody. Association with hemophiliacs' immune status and blood component usage. *Journal of the American Medical Association* 253:3409–3415, 1985.

CDC. Changing patterns of acquired immunodeficiency syndrome in hemophiliac patients—United States. *Morbidity and Mortality Weekly Report* 34:241–243, 1985.

79.

Goldsmith, J., Mosely, P., Monick, M., et al. T-lymphocyte subpopulation abnormalities in apparently healthy patients with hemophilia. *Annals of Internal Medicine* 98:294–296, 1983.

Levine, P. The acquired immunodeficiency syndrome in persons with hemophilia. *Annals of Internal Medicine* 103:723–726, 1985.

Kreiss, J., Kitchen, L., Prince, H., et al. Human T-cell leukemia virus type III antibody, lymphadenopathy, and acquired immune deficiency syndrome in hemophiliac subjects: results of a prospective study. *The American Journal of Medicine* 80:345–350, 1986.

80.

National Hemophilia Foundation Medical and Scientific Advisory Council Recommendations Concerning AIDS and Therapy of Hemophilia (revised October 13, 1984). New York: National Hemophilia Foundation, 1984.

CDC. Update: acquired immunodeficiency syndrome (AIDS) in persons with hemophilia. *Morbidity and Mortality Weekly Report* 33:589–591, 1984.

Petricciani, J., McDougal, J.S., Evatt, B. Case for concluding that heat-treated, licensed anti-haemophiliac factor is free from HTLV-III. *Lancet* 2:890–891, 1985.

Levy, J., Mitra, G., Wong, M. et al. Inactivation by wet and dry heat of AIDS-associated retroviruses during factor VIII purification from plasma. *Lancet* 1:1456–1457, 1985.

Prince, A., Horowitz, B., Brotman, B. Sterilisation of hepatitis and HTLV-III viruses by exposure to tri(n-butyl) phosphate and sodium cholate. *Lancet* 1:706–710, 1986.

81.

CDC. The safety of hepatitis B virus vaccine. *Morbidity and Mortality Weekly Report* 32:134–136, 1983.

CDC. Hepatitis B vaccine: evidence confirming lack of AIDS transmission. *Morbidity and Mortality Weekly Report* 33:685–687, 1984.

Nightingale, S. From the FDA. Hepatitis B vaccine. *Journal of the American Medical Association* 255:76, 1986.

82.

CDC. Safety of therapeutic immune globulin preparations with respect to transmission of HTLV-III/lymphadenopathy-associated virus infection. *Morbidity and Mortality Weekly Report* 35:231–233, 1986.

Wood, C., Williams, A., McNamara, J., et al. Antibody against the human immunodeficiency virus in commercial intravenous gammaglobulin preparations. *Annals of Internal Medicine* 105:536–538, 1986.

83.

Curt, G. Katterhagen, G., Mahaney, F. Immunoaugmentive therapy. A primer on the perils of unproved treatments. *Journal of the American Medical Association* 505–507, 1986.

CDC. Isolation of human T-lymphotropic virus type III/lymphadenopathy-associated virus from serum proteins given to cancer patients—Bahamas. *Morbidity and Mortality Weekly Report* 43(3):489–491, 1985.

84.

Jarlais, D., Friedman, S., Hopkins, W. Risk reduction for the acquired immunodeficiency syndrome among intravenous drug users. *Annals of Internal Medicine* 103:755–759, 1985.

Peterman, T., Jaffe, H., Feorino, P., et al. Transfusion associated acquired immunodeficiency syndrome in the United States. *Journal of the American Medical Association* 254(20):2913–2917, 1985.

Feorino, P., Jaffee, H., Palmer, E., et al. Transfusion-associated acquired immunodeficiency syndrome. Evidence for persistent infection in blood donors. *The New England Journal of Medicine* 312:1293–1296, 1985.

Jett, J., Kuritsky, J., Katzmann, J., et al. Acquired immunodeficiency syndrome associated with blood-product transfusions. *Annals of Internal Medicine* 99:621–624, 1983.

85.

From the FDA. Revised AIDS blood donor recommendations. *Journal of the American Medical Association* 257:1289, 1987.

CDC. Additional recommendations to reduce sexual and drug abuse-related transmission of human T-lymphotropic virus type III/Lymphadenopathy-associated virus. *Morbidity and Mortality Weekly Report* 35:10, 1986.

86.

Osterholm, M., Bowman, R., Chopek, M., et al. Screening donated blood and plasma for HTLV-III antibody. *The New England Journal of Medicine* 312: 1185–1188, 1985.

Fear of AIDS linked to nation's low blood supply. *Internal Medicine News* p. 44, March 1–16, 1986.

87.

Curran, J. The epidemiology and prevention of the acquired immunodeficiency syndrome. *Annals of Internal Medicine* 103:657–662, 1985.

Chamberland, M., Castro, K., Haverkos, H., et al. Acquired immunodeficiency syndrome in the United States: an analysis of cases outside high-incidence groups. *Annals of Internal Medicine* 101:617–623, 1985.

Redfield, R., Markham, P., Salahuddin, S., et al. Heterosexually acquired HTLV-III/LAV disease (AIDS-related complex and AIDS). Epidemiological evidence for female-to-male transmission. *Journal of the American Medical Association* 254:2094–2096, 1985.

88.

Slawson, S. Insect-borne transmission of AIDS? (Questions and Answers). *Journal of the American Medical Association* 254(8):1085, 1985.

Blaser, M. Insect-borne transmission of AIDS (letter). *Journal of the American Medical Association* 255(4):463, 1986.

Drotman, D.P. Reply to: insect-borne transmission of AIDS (letter). *Journal of the American Medical Association* 255(4):464, 1986.

Zuckerman, A.J. AIDS and insects (editorial). *British Medical Journal* 292:1094–1095, 1986.

Lyons, S., Jupp, P., Schoub, B. Survival of HIV in the common bedbug (letter). *Lancet* 2:45, 1986.

89.
Leads from MMWR. Acquired immunodeficiency syndrome (AIDS) in Western Palm Beach County, Florida. *Journal of the American Medical Association* 256:2936–2940, 1986.

90.
Pape, J., Liautaud, B., Thomas, F., et al. Characteristics of the acquired immunodeficiency syndrome (AIDS) in Haiti *The New England Journal of Medicine* 309:945–950 1983.

Pitchenik, A., Fischl, M., Dickenson, G., et al. Opportunistic infections and Kaposi's sarcoma among Haitians: evidence of a new acquired immunodeficiency state. *Annals of Internal Medicine* 98:277–284, 1983.

Frank, E., Weiss, J., Compas, J., et al. AIDS in Haitian Americans: a reassessment. *Cancer Research* 45:4619s–4620s, 1985.

91.
Weiss, S.H., Goedert, J., Sarngadharan, M., et al. Screening test for HTLV-III (AIDS agent) antibodies. *Journal of the American Medical Association* 254:221–225, 1985.

Marwick, C. Blood banks give HTLV-III test positive appraisal at five months. *Journal of the American Medical Association* 254(13):1681–1683, 1985.

Osterholm, M., Bowman, R., Chopek, M., et al. Screening donated blood and plasma for HTLV-III antibody. Facing more than one crisis? *The New England Journal of Medicine* 312(18):1185–1188, 1985.

92.

CDC. Provisional Public Health Service inter-agency recommendations for screening donated blood and plasma for antibody to the virus causing acquired immunodeficiency syndrome. *Morbidity and Mortality Weekly Report* 34:1–4, 1985.

Osterholm, M., Bowman, R., Chopek, M., et al. Screening donated blood and plasma for HTLV-III antibody. Facing more than one crisis? *The New England Journal of Medicine* 312(18):1185–1188, 1985.

93.

CDC. Provisional Public Health Service inter-agency recommendations for screening donated blood and plasma for antibody to the virus causing acquired immunodeficiency syndrome. *Morbidity and Mortality Weekly Report* 34:1–4, 1985.

94.

Mason, J. Alternative sites for screening blood for antibodies to AIDS virus. *The New England Journal of Medicine* 313(18):1157–1158, 1985.

CDC. HTLV-III/LAV antibody testing at alternative sites. *Morbidity and Mortality Weekly Report* 35:284–287, 1986.

95.

CDC. Update: Public Health Service workshop on human T-lymphotropic virus type III antibody testing—United States. *Morbidity and Mortality Weekly Report* 34:477–478, 1985.

96.

Petricciani, J. Licensed tests for antibody to human T-lymphotropic virus type III. Sensitivity and specificity. *Annals of Internal Medicine* 103:726–729, 1985.

CDC. Results of human T-lymphotropic virus type III test kits reported from blood collection centers—United States, April 22–May 19, 1985. *Morbidity and Mortality Weekly Report* 34(25):375–376, 1985.

Osterholm, M., Bowman, R., Chopek, M., et al. Screening donated blood and plasma for HTLV-III antibody. Facing more than one crisis? *The New England Journal of Medicine* 312(18):1185–1188, 1985.

Mendenhall, C., Roselle, G., Grossman, C., et al. False positive tests for HTLV-III antibodies in alcoholic patients with hepatitis. *The New England Journal of Medicine* 314:921–922, 1986.

97.

CDC. Update: Public Health Service workshop on human T-lymphotropic virus type III antibody testing—United States. *Morbidity and Mortality Weekly Report* 34:477–478, 1985.

Ward, J., Grindon, A., Feorino, P., et al. Laboratory and epidemiologic evaluation of an enzyme immunoassay for antibodies to HTLV-III. *Journal of the American Medical Association* 256:357–361, 1986.

98–99.

CDC. Update: Public Health Service workshop on human T-lymphotropic virus type III antibody testing—United States. *Morbidity and Mortality Weekly Report* 34:477–478, 1985.

Esteban, J., Shih, J., Tai, C., et al. Importance of Western blot analysis in predicting infectivity of anti-HTLV-III/LAV positive blood. *Lancet* 2:1083–1086, 1985.

100.

Assume population A where the incidence of AIDS is 1 in 500 persons and population B where the incidence is 1 in 50,000 persons. Consider that an antibody test finds incorrectly that 1 out of 5,000 normal people are antibody positive. Then, in population A, of every 50,000 persons tested, 100 will be correctly diagnosed as having antibody positivity [1/500 = x/50,000] and 10 persons will be diagnosed incorrectly [1/5000 = x/50,000] for an accuracy of about 90 percent. In population B, of 50,000 persons tested, the low incidence of antibody positivity in the population would result in only 1 diagnosis of antibody positivity [1/50,000 = x/50,000]. However, about 10 individuals would be incorrectly diagnosed as having antibody positivity [1/5000 = x/50,000] for an accuracy of about 10 percent.

Carlson, J., Bryant, M., Hinrichs, S., et al. AIDS serology testing in low- and high-risk groups. *Journal of the American Medical Association* 253(23):3405–3408, 1985.

Barry, M., Mulley, A., Singer, D. Screening for HTLV-III antibodies: the relation between prevalence and positive predictive value and its social consequences (letter). *Journal of the American Medical Association* 253(23):3395–3396, 1985.

01.

Salahuddin, S., Groopman, J., Markham, P., et al. HTLV-III in symptom-free seronegative persons. *Lancet* 2:1418–1420, 1984.

Anonymous. Needlestick transmission of HTLV-III from a patient infected in Africa. *Lancet* 2:1376–1377, 1984.

CDC. Apparent transmission of human T-lymphotropic virus type III/lymphadenopathy-associated virus from child to mother providing health care. *Morbidity and Mortality Weekly Report* 35:5, 1986.

02.

CDC. Provisional Public Health Service inter-agency recommendations for screening donated blood and plasma for antibody to the virus causing acquired immunodeficiency syndrome. *Morbidity and Mortality Weekly Report* 34:1–4, 1985.

Ho, D., Schooley, R., Rota, T., et al. HTLV-III in the semen and blood of a healthy homosexual man. *Science* 226:451–453, 1984.

Salahuddin, S., Groopman, J., Markham, P., et al. HTLV-III in symptom-free seronegative persons. *Lancet* 2:1418–1420, 1984.

03.

Wong-Staal, F., Gallo, R. Human T-lymphotropic viruses. *Nature* 317:395–403, 1985.

Sarngadharan, M., Popovic, M., Bruch, L., et al. Antibodies reactive with human T-lymphotropic retrovirus (HTLV-III) in the serum of patients with AIDS. *Science* 224:506–508, 1984.

Biggar, R., Melbye, M., Ebbesen, P., et al. HTLV-III antibody variation in AIDS and AIDS-risk homosexual men: decline prior to onset of AIDS-related illness. *British Medical Journal* 1985 (in press).

Marwick, C. Blood banks give HTLV-III test positive appraisal at five months. *Journal of the American Medical Association* 254(13):1681–1683, 1985.

104.

Salahuddin, S., Groopman, J., Markham, P., et al. HTLV-III in symptom-free seronegative persons. *Lancet* 2:1418–1420, 1984.

Ho, D., Schooley, R., Rota, T., et al. HTLV-III in the semen and blood of a healthy homosexual man. *Science* 226:451–453, 1984.

CDC. Leads from the MMWR. Transfusion-associated human T-lymphotropic virus type III/lymphadenopathy-associated virus infection from a seronegative donor—Colorado *Journal of the American Medical Association* 256:574–575, 1986.

105.

CDC. World Health Organization workshop: conclusions and recommendations on acquired immunodeficiency syndrome. *Morbidity and Mortality Weekly Report* 34:275–277, 1985.

AIDS update. *American Medical News,* March 7, 1986, p 28.

Saag, M., Britz, J. Limitations of testing: asymptomatic blood donor with a false positive HTLV-III Western blot. *The New England Journal of Medicine* 314:118, 1986.

106.

Screening for AIDS. *Medical Letter* 27:29–30, 1985.

Salahuddin, S., et al. HTLV-III in symptom-free seronegative persons. *Lancet* 2:1418–1420, 1984.

Mayer, K., Stoddard, A., McCusker, J., et al. Human T-lymphotropic virus type III in high risk antibody negative homosexual men. *Annals of Internal Medicine* 104:194–196, 1986.

107.

CDC. Provisional Public Health Service inter-agency recommendations for screening donated blood and plasma for antibody to the virus causing acquired immunodeficiency syndrome. *Morbidity and Mortality Weekly Report* 34:1–4, 1985.

Salahuddin, S., Groopman, J., Markham, P., et al. HTLV-III in sympton-free seronegative persons. *Lancet* 2:1418–1420, 1984.

108.

Curran, J. The epidemiology and prevention of the acquired immunodeficiency syndrome. *Annals of Internal Medicine* 103:657–662, 1985.

Gendelman, H., Phelps, W., Feigenbaum, L., et al. Trans-activation of the human immunodeficiency virus terminal repeat sequence by DNA viruses. *Proceedings of the National Academy of Sciences* 83:9759–9763, 1986.

Fauci, A. Current issues in developing a strategy for dealing with the acquired immunodeficiency syndrome. *Proceedings of the National Academy of Sciences* 83:9278–9283, 1986.

109.

Blattner, W., Biggar, R., Weiss, S., et al. Epidemiology of human T-lymphotropic virus type III and the risk of the acquired immunodeficiency syndrome. *Annals of Internal Medicine* 103:665–670, 1985.

AIDS antibody testing: what does a positive result mean? *Data Centrum* 2:18–24, 1985.

Francis, D., Jaffe, J., Fultz, P., et al. The natural history of infection with the lymphadenopathy-associated virus/human T-lymphotropic virus type III. *Annals of Internal Medicine* 103:719–722, 1985.

110.

Eales, L-J, Nye, K., Parkin, J., et al. Association of different allelic forms of group specific component with susceptibility to and clinical manifestation of human immunodeficiency virus infection. *Lancet,* pp. 999–1002, 1987.

111.

CDC. Additional recommendations to reduce sexual and drug abuse-related transmission of human T-lymphotropic virus type III/lymphadenopathy-associated virus. *Morbidity and Mortality Weekly Report* 35:10, 1986.

Francis, D., Chin, J. The prevention of acquired immunodeficiency syndrome in the United States: an objective strategy for medicine, public health, business, and the community. *Journal of the American Medical Association* 257:1357–1366, 1987.

112.

CDC. Recommendations for assisting in the prevention of perinatal transmission of HTLV-III/LAV and acquired immunodeficiency syndrome. *Morbidity and Mortality Weekly Report* 34:721–731, 1985.

113.

Ibid.

Bass, M., Molloshok, R. In Guttmacher, A.F., Rovinsky, J. (eds.). *Medical, Surgical and Gynecological Complications of Pregnancy.* Baltimore: Williams & Williams, p. 526, 1960.

Siegel, M., Goldberg, M. Incidence of poliomyelitis in pregnancy. *The New England Journal of Medicine* 253:841–843, 1955.

Scott, G., Fischl, M., Klimas, N., et al. Mothers of infants with the acquired immunodeficiency syndrome: evidence for both symptomatic and asymptomatic carriers. *Journal of the American Medical Association* 253:363–366, 1985.

Weinberg, E.D. Pregnancy-associated depression of cell-mediated immunity. *Review of Infectious Diseases* 6:814–831, 1984.

114.

Lundberg, G. The age of AIDS: a great time for defensive living. *Journal of the American Medical Association* 253:3440–3441, 1985.

115.

CDC. Tuberculosis—United States, 1985 and possible impact of human T-lymphotropic virus type III/lymphadenopathy-associated virus infection. *Morbidity and Mortality Weekly Report* 35:5, 1986.

CDC. Diagnosis and management of mycobacterial infection and disease in persons with human T-lymphotropic virus type III/lymphadenopathy-associated virus infection. *Morbidity and Mortality Weekly Report* 35:448–451, 1986.

Melbye, M., Biggar, R., Ebbersen, P., et al. Long-term seropositivity for human T-lymphotropic virus type III in homosexual men without the acquired immunodeficiency syndrome: development of immunological and clinical abnormalities. *Annals of Internal Medicine* 104:496–500, 1986.

116.
Staver, S. Nation's AIDS epidemic triggers insurance woes for millions of people. *American Medical News* pp. 1–39, April 11, 1986.

No insurance denial if at risk for AIDS. *Internal Medicine News,* p. 2, August 1–14, 1986.

AIDS: Employers' Rights and Responsibilities. Chicago: Commerce Clearing House, 1985 (4025 W. Peterson Avenue, Chicago, IL 60646).

117.
CDC. Provisional Public Health Service inter-agency recommendations for screening donated blood and plasma for antibody to the virus causing acquired immunodeficiency syndrome. *Morbidity and Mortality Weekly Report* 34:1–4, 1985.

CDC. Heterosexual transmission of human T-lymphotropic virus type III/lymphadenopathy-associated virus. *Morbidity and Mortality Weekly Report* 34:561–562, 1985.

D'Agulla, R., Williams, A., Kleber, H., et al. Prevalence of HTLV-III infection among New Haven, Connecticut parental drug abusers in 1982–1983. *The New England Journal of Medicine* 314:117, 1986.

CDC. Recommendations for assisting in the prevention of perinatal transmission of human T-lymphotropic virus type III/lymphadenopathy-associated virus and acquired immunodeficiency syndrome. *Morbidity and Mortality Weekly Report* 34:721–732, 1985.

Kreiss, J., Koech, D., Plummer, F., et al. AIDS virus infection in Nairobi prostitutes. *The New England Journal of Medicine* 314:414–418, 1986.

Robertson, J., Bucknall, A., Welsby, P., et al. Epidemic of AIDS related virus (HTLV-III/LAV) infection among intravenous drug abusers. *British Medical Journal* 292:527–529, 1986.

Ragni, M., Tegmeier, G., Levy, J., et al. AIDS retrovirus antibodies in hemophiliacs treated with factor VIII or factor IX concentrates, cryoprecipitate, or fresh frozen plasma: prevalence, seroconversion rate, and clinical correlations. *Blood* 67:592–595, 1986.

Kalish, R., Cable, R., Roberts, S. Voluntary deferral of blood and HTLV-III antibody positivity. *The New England Journal of Medicine* 314:1115–1116, 1986.

118.
Older soldiers more likely to carry HTLV-III antibody. *American Medical News,* p. 59, April 11, 1986.

CDC. Human T-lymphotropic virus type III/lymphadenopathy-associated virus antibody prevalence in U.S. military recruit applicants. *Morbidity and Mortality Weekly Report* 35:412–423, 1986.

Krieger, L. Pentagon expanding testing: all military personnel face AIDS screening. *American Medical News,* p. 10, November 1, 1985.

Redfield, R., Markham, P., Salahuddin, S., et al. Heterosexually acquired HTLV-III/LAV disease (AIDS-related complex and AIDS). Epidemiological evidence for female-to-male transmission. *Journal of the American Medical Association* 254:2094–2096, 1985.

119.
CDC. Testing donors of organs, tissues, and semen for antibody to human T-lymphotropic virus type-III/lymphadenopathy-associated virus. *Morbidity and Mortality Weekly Report* 34:294, 1985.

CDC. Additional recommendations to reduce sexual and drug abuse-related transmission of human T-lymphotropic virus type III/lymphadenopathy-associated virus. *Morbidity and Mortality Weekly Report* 35:10, 1986.

120.
CDC. Declining rates of rectal and pharyngeal gonorrhea among males—New York City. *Morbidity and Mortality Weekly Report* 3:295–297, 1984.

Lundberg, G. The age of AIDS: a great time for defensive living (editorial). *Journal of the American Medical Association* 253(23):3440–3441, 1985.

Handsfield, H. Decreasing incidence of gonorrhea in homosexually active men—minimal effect on risk of AIDS. *Western Journal of Medicine* 143:469–470, 1985.

Conant, M., Hardy, D., Sernatinger, J., et al. Condoms prevent transmission of the AIDS-associated retrovirus. *Journal of the American Medical Association* 255:1706, 1986.

121.
Assume 33 percent of one's random sexual contacts are antibody positive for the AIDS virus. Then, assuming 40 sexual contacts, the risk of coming into contact with at least one of these persons with antibody positive results would be $1.0-[2/3]^{40}$ or approximately 100 percent. Assuming only four sexual contacts, the risk would only be lowered to $1.0-[2/3]^4$ or 81 percent.

Handsfield, H. Decreasing incidence of gonorrhea in homosexually active men—minimal effect on risk of AIDS. *Western Journal of Medicine* 143:469–470, 1985.

122.
CDC. Self-reported behavioral changes among homosexual and bisexual men—San Francisco. *Morbidity and Mortality Weekly Report* 40:613–615, 1985.

123.
Conant, M., Hardy, D., Sernatinger, J., et al. Condoms prevent transmission of AIDS-associated retrovirus (letter). *Journal of the American Medical Association* 255:1706, 1986.

Hicks, D., Martin, L., Getchell, J., et al. Inactivation of

HTLV-III/LAV infected cultures of normal human lymphocytes by nonoxynol-9 in vitro. *Lancet* 2:1422–1423, 1985.

Stone, K., Grimes, D., Magder, L. Primary prevention of sexually transmitted diseases: a primer for clinicians. *Journal of the American Medical Association* 255:1763–1766, 1986.

124.

Peterman T., Curran J. Sexual transmission of human immunodeficiency virus. *Journal of the American Medical Association* 256:2222–2226, 1986.

125.

Weiss, S., Saxinger, W., Rechtman, D., et al. HTLV-III infection among health care workers. Association with needlestick injuries. *Journal of the American Medical Association* 254(15):2089–2096, 1985.

CDC. Update: evaluation of human T-lymphotropic virus type III/lymphadenopathy-associated virus infection in healthcare personnel—United States. *Morbidity and Mortality Weekly Report* 34:575–577, 1985.

CDC. Recommendations for preventing transmission of infection with human T-lymphotropic virus type III/lymphadenopathy-associated virus in the workplace. *Morbidity and Mortality Weekly Report* 34:681–695, 1985.

Stricof, R., Morse, D. HTLV-III/LAV seroconversion following a deep intramuscular needlestick injury. *The New England Journal of Medicine* 314:1115, 1986.

126.

CDC. Apparent transmission of human T-lymphotropic virus type III/lymphadenopathy-associated virus from child to mother providing health care. *Morbidity and Mortality Weekly Report* 35:5, 1986.

127.

CDC. Recommendations for preventing transmission of infection with human T-lymphotropic virus type III/ lymphadenopathy-associated virus in the workplace. *Morbidity and Mortality Weekly Report* 34:681–695, 1985.

CDC. Recommendations for preventing transmission of infection with human T-lymphotropic virus type III/

lymphadenopathy-associated virus during invasive procedures. *Morbidity and Mortality Weekly Report* 35:221–223, 1986.

128.
Ibid.

129.
Recovery of HTLV-III from contact lenses. *Lancet* 1:379–380, 1986.

CDC. Recommendations for preventing possible transmission of human T-lymphotropic virus type III/lymphadenopathy-associated virus from tears. *Morbidity and Mortality Weekly Report* 34:533–534, 1985.

130.
The California and Wisconsin laws prohibiting employees and others from undergoing nonvoluntary AIDS antibody testing are described in *AIDS: Employers' Rights and Responsibilities.* Chicago: Commerce Clearing House, pp. 42–43, 1985 (4025 W. Peterson Avenue, Chicago, IL 60646).

AIDS Update. The lambda report on AIDS-related legal issues. 1, p. 5, December 1985.

131.
Saviteer, S., White, G., Cohen, M., et al. HTLV-III exposure during cardiopulmonary resuscitation. *The New England Journal of Medicine* 313:1606–1607, 1985.

CDC. Recommendations for preventing transmission of infection with human T-lymphotropic virus type III/lymphadenopathy-associated virus in the workplace. *Morbidity and Mortality Weekly Report* 34:681–694, 1985.

132.
Ibid.

133.
Ibid.

134.
Stewart, G., Cunningham, A., Driscoll, G., et al. Transmission of human T-cell lymphotropic virus type III (HTLV-III) by artificial insemination by donor. *Lancet* 2:581–583, 1985.

Mascola, L., Guinan, M. Screening to reduce transmission of sexually transmitted diseases in semen used for artificial insemination. *The New England Journal of Medicine* 314:1354–1359, 1986.

135.

Martin, L., McDougal, J., Loskoski, S. Disinfection and inactivation of the human T-lymphotropic virus type III/lymphadenopathy-associated virus. *Journal of Infectious Disease* 152:400–403, 1985.

CDC. Recommendations for preventing transmission of infection with human T-lymphotropic virus type III/lymphadenopathy-associated virus in the workplace. *Morbidity and Mortality Weekly Report* 34:681–694, 1985.

Resnick, L., Veren, K., Salahuddin, S., et al. Stability and inactivation of HTLV-III/LAV under clinical and laboratory environments. *Journal of the American Medical Association* 255:1887–1891, 1986.

136.

Shafer, R., Offit, K., Macris, N., et al. Possible risk of steroid administration in patients at risk for AIDS. *Lancet* 1:934–935, 1985.

Real, F., Krown, S., Koziner, B. Steroid-related development of Kaposi's sarcoma in a homosexual man with Burkitt's lymphoma. *The American Journal of Medicine* 80:119–122, 1986.

Markham, P., Salahuddin, S., Veren, K., et al. Hydrocortisone and some other hormones enhance the expression of HTLV-III. *International Journal of Cancer* 37:67–72, 1986.

Chlebowski, R. Significance of altered nutritional status in acquired immune deficiency syndrome (AIDS). *Nutrition and Cancer* 7:85–91, 1985.

137.

Conte, J., Hadley, W.K., Sande, M. Special report. Infection control guidelines for patients with the acquired immunodeficiency syndrome (AIDS). *The New England Journal of Medicine* 309(12):740–744, 1983.

Ray, C.G. Cytomegalic inclusion disease (salivary gland virus disease). In Isselbacher, K., Adams, R., Braunwald, E., et al. (eds.). *Harrison's Principles of Internal Medicine*. (9th ed.). New York: McGraw Hill, pp.852–854, 1980.

138.
Prompt, C., Reis, M., Grillo, F., et al. Transmission of AIDS virus at renal transplantation. *Lancet* 2:672, 1985.

CDC. Testing donors of organs, tissues, and semen for antibody to human T-lymphotropic virus type III/lymphadenopathy-associated virus. *Morbidity and Mortality Weekly Report* 34:294, 1985.

L'Age-Stehr, J., Schwartz, A., Offermann, G. HTLV-III infection in kidney transplant recipients. *Lancet* 2:1361–1362, 1985.

139.
Quinn, T., Mann, J., Curran, J., et al. AIDS in Africa: an epidemiological paradigm. *Science* 234:955–963, 1986.

140.
Gallo, R., Salahuddin, S., Popovic, M., et al. Frequent detection and isolation of cytopathic retroviruses (HTLV-III) from patients with AIDS and at risk for AIDS. *Science* 224:500–503, 1984.

Levy, J., Hoffman, A., Kramer, S., et al. Isolation of lymphocytopathic retroviruses from San Francisco patients with AIDS. *Science* 225:840–843, 1984.

Sarngadharan, M., Popovic, M., Bruch, M., et al. Antibodies reactive with human T-lymphotropic retroviruses (HTLV-III) in the serum of patients with AIDS. *Science* 224:506–508, 1984.

Zagury, D., Bernard, J., Leibowitch, J., et al. HTLV-III in cells cultured from semen of two patients with AIDS. *Science* 226:449–451, 1984.

Ho, H.D., Schooley, R., Rota, T., et al. HTLV-III in the semen and blood of a healthy homosexual man. *Science* 226:451–453, 1984.

Groopman, J., Salahuddin, S., Sarngadharan, M., et al. HTLV-III in saliva of people with AIDS-related complex and healthy homosexual men at risk for AIDS. *Science* 226:447–449, 1984.

Curran, J., The epidemiology and prevention of the acquired immunodeficiency syndrome. *Annals of Internal Medicine* 103:657–662, 1985.

Fazakerly, J., Webb, H. Isolation of AIDS virus from cell-free breast milk of three healthy virus carriers. *Lancet* 2:891–892, 1985.

Vogt, M., Witt, D., Craven, D., et al. Isolation of HTLV-III/LAV from cervical secretions of women at risk for AIDS. *Lancet* 1:525–527, 1986.

CDC. Recommendations for preventing possible transmission of human T-lymphotropic virus type III/lymphadenopathy-associated virus from tears. *Morbidity and Mortality Weekly Report* 34:533–534, 1985.

141.
CDC. Education and foster care of children infected with human T-lymphotropic virus type III/lymphadenopathy-associated virus. *Morbidity and Mortality Weekly Report* 34:517–521, 1985.

American Academy of Pediatrics. School attendance of children and adolescents with human T-lymphotropic virus III/lymphadenopathy-associated virus infection. *Pediatrics* 77:430–432, 1986.

142.
Physicians named to NY panel to decide AIDS schooling cases. *American Medical News,* p. 31, October 11, 1985.

School, health officials respond to AIDS concerns. *American Medical News,* p. 2, October 18, 1985.

Teen with AIDS can return to classroom under ruling. *American Medical News,* pp. 20–21, December 13, 1985.

143–144.
Health and Public Policy Committee, American College of Physicians and the Infectious Diseases Society of America Position paper: acquired immunodeficiency syndrome *Annals of Internal Medicine* 104:575–581, 1986.

145.

Different statures relevant to discrimination against persons with AIDS are reviewed in the excellent article by Leonard, A.S. Employment discrimination against persons with AIDS. *Dayton Law Review* 10(3):681–702, 1985.

AIDS: Employers' Rights and Responsibilities. Chicago: Commerce Clearing House, 1985 (4025 W. Peterson Avenue, Chicago, IL 60646).

146–148.

Matthews, G., Neslund, V. The initial impact of AIDS on public health law in the United States—1986. *Journal of the American Medical Association* 257:344–352, 1987.

AIDS: Employers' Rights and Responsibilities. Chicago: Commerce Clearing House, 1985 (4025 W. Peterson Avenue, Chicago, IL 60646).

AIDS Legal Guide: A Professional Resource on AIDS-Related Issues and Discrimination. 1986 (Available from LAMBDA Legal Defense and Education Fund, 666 Broadway, New York, NY 10012).

150.

Foege, W. Public health and preventative medicine. *Journal of the American Medical Association* 254(16):2330–2332, 1985.

151.

Brunet, J., Ancelle, R. The international occurrence of the acquired immunodeficiency syndrome. *Annals of Internal Medicine* 103:670–674, 1985.

CDC. Update: acquired immunodeficiency syndrome—Europe. *Morbidity and Mortality Weekly Report* 35(3):35–44, 1986.

Soviets admit AIDS cases. *Nature* 318:502, 1985.

Quinn, T., Mann, J., Curran, J., et al. AIDS in Africa: an epidemiological paradigm. *Science* 234:955–963, 1986.

152.

Ibid.

WHO. Acquired immunodeficiency syndrome (AIDS). Report

on the situation in Europe as of 31 December 1984. *Weekly Epidemiological Record* 60:85–92, 1985.

Mann, J., Francis, H., Quinn, T., et al. Surveillance for AIDS in a central African city. Kinshasa, Zaire. *Journal of the American Medical Association* 255:3255–3257, 1986.

153–156.
Quinn, T., Mann, J., Curran, J., et al. AIDS in Africa: an epidemiological paradigm. *Science* 234:955–963, 1986.

Biggar, R. The AIDS problem in Africa. *Lancet* 1:79–82, 1986.

Clumeck, N., Robert-Guroff, M., Van De Perre, P., et al. Seroepidemiological studies of HTLV-III antibody prevalence among selected groups of heterosexual Africans. *Journal of the American Medical Association* 254(18):2599–2608, 1985.

Mann, J., Francis, H., Quinn, T., et al. Surveillance for AIDS in a central Africa city, Kinshasa, Zaire. *Journal of the American Medical Association* 255:3255–3259, 1986.

157.
World Health Organization announces war on AIDS. *American Medical News*, p. 13, October 4, 1985.

Restrictions set on blood donation. *American Medical News,* p. 13, October 4, 1985.

AIDS cases, fear rising in Asian countries. *American Medical News*, p. 26, October 25, 1985.

Acquired immunodeficiency syndrome in Saudi Arabia. The American-Saudi connection. *Journal of the American Medical Association* 255:383–384, 1986.

158.
Curran, J., Morgan, W., Hardy, A., et al. The epidemiolog of AIDS: current status and future prospects. *Scienc* 229:1352–1357, 1985.

Public fears about AIDS continue to grow. *American Medica News,* p. 20, January 3, 1986.

159.
Curran, J., Morgan, W., Hardy, A., et al. The epidemiolog

of AIDS: current status and future prospects. *Science* 229:1352–1357, 1985.

CDC. Recommendations for assisting in the prevention of perinatal transmission of HTLV-III/LAV and acquired immunodeficiency syndrome. *Morbidity and Mortality Weekly Report* 34:721–731, 1985.

Leads from the MMWR. CDC. Update: acquired immunodeficiency syndrome—United States. *Journal of the American Medical Association* 255:593–598, 1986.

60.

Kristal, A. The impact of the acquired immunodeficiency syndrome on patterns of premature death in New York City. *Journal of the American Medical Association* 255:2306–2310, 1986.

61.

Leads from the MMWR. CDC. Update: acquired immundeficiency syndrome—United States. *Journal of the American Medical Association* 255:593–598, 1986.

Surgeon General's Report on Acquired Immune Deficiency Syndrome. (November 1986). (Available from the United States Public Health Service, AIDS, Box 14252, Washington, DC 20044).

Osborn, J. The AIDS epidemic: an overview of the science. *Issues in Science and Technology,* pp. 39–55, Winter 1986.

Confronting AIDS: Directions for Public Health, Health Care, and Research. Washington, DC: National Academy Press, 1986 (2101 Constitution Avenue, NW, Washington, DC 20418).

62.

Landesman, S., Ginzbug, H., Weiss, S. The AIDS epidemic. *The New England Journal of Medicine* 312:521–524, 1985.

AIDS costs battering hospitals. *American Medical News,* p. 2, November 15, 1985.

163.

Outpatient AIDS care gets financial boost. *Medical World News*, p. 24, March 4, 1986.

AIDS patients need more nursing time. *American Medical News*, p. 30, March 21, 1986.

164.

$244 million approved for efforts to fight AIDS. *Internal Medicine News*, p. 2, February 1–16, 1986.

Confronting AIDS: Directions for Public Health, Health Care, and Research. Washington, DC: National Academy Press, 1986. (2101 Constitution Avenue, NW, Washington, DC 20418).

165.

Ibid.

166.

Budget of the United States Government: Fiscal Year 1986 Washington DC: U.S. Government Printing Office, IK1–IK7, 1985.

167.

Hirsch, M., Kaplan, J. Prospects of therapy for infection with human T-lymphotropic virus type III. *Annals of Internal Medicine* 103:750–755, 1985.

Antivirals. *FDA Drug Bulletin* 15:30–31, 1985.

Broder, S., Collins, J., Markham, P., et al. Effects of suramin on HTLV-III/LAV infection presenting as Kaposi's sarcoma or AIDS-related complex: clinical pharmacology and suppression of virus replication in vivo. *Lancet* 2:627–630, 1985.

Levine, A., Gill, P., Cohen, J., et al. Suramin antiviral therapy in the acquired immunodeficiency syndrome: clinical, immunologic, and virologic results. *Annals of Internal Medicine* 105:32–37, 1986.

Sarin, P., Gallo, R., Scheer, D., et al. Effects of a novel compound (AL 721) on HTLV-III infectivity in vitro. *The New England Journal of Medicine* 313:1289–1290, 1985

Yarchoan, R., Weinhold, K., Lyerly, H., et al. Administration of 3'-azido-3'-deoxythymidine, an inhibitor of HTLV-II

LAV replication, to patients with AIDS or AIDS-related complex. *Lancet* 1:575–580, 1986.

AIDS therapy must cross blood/brain barrier. *Internal Medicine News,* p. 64, February 1–14, 1986.

68.

From the Food and Drug Administration. AZT Available Under AIDS Treatment Protocol. *Journal of the American Medical Association* 256:2657, 1986.

69.

Riesenberg, D. Anti-AIDS agents show varying early results in vitro and in vivo. *Journal of the American Medical Association* 254:2521–2529, 1985.

Antivirals. *FDA Drug Bulletin* 15:30–31, 1985.

70.

Riesenberg, D. Anti-AIDS agents show varying early results in vitro and in vivo. *Journal of the American Medical Association* 254(18):2521–2529, 1985.

71.

Curran, J., Morgan, W., Hardy, A., et al. The epidemiology of AIDS: current status and future prospects. *Science* 229:1352–1357, 1985.

72.

Letvin, N., Daniel, M., Schgal, P., et al. Induction of AIDS-like disease in macaque monkeys with T-cell tropic retrovirus STLV-III. *Science* 230:71–73, 1985.

Power, M., Marx, P., Bryant, M., et al. Nucleotide sequence of SRV-1, a type D simian acquired immune deficiency syndrome retrovirus. *Science* 231:1567–1572, 1986.

Fisher, A., Feinberg, M., Josephs, S., et al. The *trans*-activator gene of HTLV-III is essential for virus replication. *Nature* 1(320):367–370, 1986.

Lee, T-H, Coligan, J., Allan, J., et al. A new HTLV-III/LAV protein encoded by a gene found in cytopathic retroviruses. *Science* 231:1546–1553, 1986.

Lan, N., Franchini, G., Wong-Staal, F., et al. Identification of HTLV-III/LAV *sor* gene product and detection of antibodies in human sera. *Science* 231:1553–1555, 1986.

Fisher, A., Ratner, L., Mitsuya, H., et al. Infectious mutants of HTLV-III with changes in the 3' region and markedly reduced cytopathic effects. *Science* 232:655–659, 1986.

173.

Riesenberg, D. Anti-AIDS agents show varying early results in vitro and in vivo. *Journal of the American Medical Association* 254:2521–2529, 1985.

Treatment of opportunistic infections and malignancies. *FDA Bulletin* 15:32, 1985.

Norman, C. News and Comment. AIDS therapy: new push for clinical trials. *Science* 230:1355–1358, 1985.

174.

Treatment of opportunistic infections and malignancies. *FDA Bulletin* 15:32, 1985.

175.

Riesenberg, D. Anti-AIDS agents show varying early results in vitro and in vivo. *Journal of the American Medical Association* 254:2521–2529, 1985.

176.

National foundation established for AIDS research. *American Medical News*, pp. 9–10, November 1, 1985.

177.

Ibid.

178.

AIDS: Employers' Rights and Responsibilities. Chicago: Commerce Clearing House, 1985 (4025 W. Peterson Avenue, Chicago, IL 60646).

179.

This list of resource centers was compiled by three groups:

- the staff of the *Journal of the American Medical Association* with the help of Dr. Alvin Novack, Yale University and Mark Behar, National Coalition of Gay STD Services (see Goldsmith, M. Many groups offer AIDS information and support. *Journal of the American Medical Association* 254:2522–2523, 1985.

- the staff of *Occupational Health and Safety* (See *Occupational Health and Safety*, pp. 28–29, April 1986.

• the Office of the Surgeon General of the United States (See *Surgeon General's Report on Acquired Immune Deficiency Syndrome*. (Available from U.S. Public Health Service, AIDS, Box 14252, Washington, DC 20044).

180.

Matthews, G., Neslund, V. The initial impact of AIDS on public health law in the United States—1985. *Journal of the American Medical Association* 257:344–352, 1987.

181.

Leads from the MMWR. Availabililty of informational material on AIDS. *Journal of the American Medical Association* 257:601, 1987.

184.

Jonsen, A., Cooke, M., Koenig, B., et al. AIDS and ethics. *Issues in Science and Technology*. pp. 56–65, Winter 1986.

AIDS: the emerging ethical dilemmas (suppl). *Hastings Center Report* 15:(4):1–32, 1985.

Matthews, G., Neslund, V. The initial impact of AIDS on public health law in the United States—1985. *Journal of the American Medical Association* 257:344–352, 1987.

185.

Jonsen, A., Cooke, M., Koenig, B., et al. AIDS and ethics. *Issues in Science and Technology*, pp. 56–65, Winter 1986.

186.

50% for quarantine. *Hospital Tribune*, p. 7, February 12, 1986.

Fear of AIDS linked to nation's low blood supply. *Internal Medicine News*, p. 44, March 1–16, 1986.

Confronting AIDS: Directions for Public Health, Health Care, and Research. Washington, DC: National Academy Press, 1986 (2101 Constitution Avenue, NW, Washington, DC 20418).

187.

Steinbrook, R., Lo, B., Moulton, J., et al. Preferences of

homosexual men with AIDS for life-sustaining treatment. *The New England Journal of Medicine* 314:457–460, 1986.

188.

Kubler-Ross, E. *AIDS: The Ultimate Challenge*. New York: Macmillan, 1987.

Elisabeth Kubler-Ross: Life, Death, and the Dying Patient. Parts I and II, 60 minutes. University of Washington: E. Kubler-Ross, 1982. (Available from The Elisabeth Kubler-Ross Center, S. Route 616, Headwaters, VA 24442)

Holland, J., Tross, S. The psychosocial and neuropsychiatric sequelae of the acquired immunodeficiency syndrome. *Annals of Internal Medicine* 103:760–764. 1985.

Nichols, S. Psychosocial reactions of persons with the acquired immunodeficiency syndrome. *Annals of Internal Medicine* 103:765–767, 1985.

189.

Marx, J. Indications of a new virus in MS patients. *Science* 230:1028, 1985.

Koprowski, H., DeFreitas, E., Harper, M., et al. Multiple sclerosis and human T-cell lymphotropic retroviruses. *Nature* 2:318–322, 1985.

Wong-Staal, F., Gallo, R. Human T-lymphotropic retroviruses. *Nature* 317:395–403, 1985.

Olsen, R., Blakesle, J., Tarr, M., et al. Association of HTLV-like antibodies and antigens in systemic lupus-erythematosus patients (abstract). *Journal of Cell Biology* S10A:195, 1986.

Price, R., Navia, B., Cho, E-S. AIDS encephalopathy. In Booss, J., Thornton, G. (eds.). Infectious Diseases of the Central Nervous System. *Neurologic Clinics* 4(1):285–301, 1986.

Barnes, D. Nervous and immune system disorders linked in a variety of diseases. *Science* 232:160–161, 1986.

Index

Note: Numbers in parentheses refer to questions where indexed material may be found.

Acquired
definition (5-7)
diseases (7)
Acquired Immunodeficiency-
Related Complex (ARC)
definition of syndrome (41)
and risk of developing AIDS
(43)
similarity to AIDS (41, 42)
Acquired Immunodeficiency
Syndrome (AIDS)
Acquired Immunodeficiency-
Related Complex and
(41-43)
Africa, role of AIDS (153-155)
antibody positivity and (*see*
Antibody)
artificial insemination and (134)
asymptomatic virus carrier and
spread of (*see* Carrier)
at risk groups (64)
attitudes of Americans (186)
Australia, prevalence in (151)
Austria, prevalence in (151)
bacterial infections and (30-32)
Belgium, prevalence in (151)
blood transfusion and (*see* Blood
transfusion)
Brazil, prevalence in (151)
Canada, prevalence in (151)
causative agent (9, 13)
children and (*see* Children)
China, prevalence in (151)
Communion as a risk factor for
(132)
condoms to reduce risk (122,
123)
date first noted in U.S. (1, 5)
definition (4, 8, 28, 40, 50)
dementia and (34)

Denmark, prevalence in (151)
diaphragms to reduce risk (123)
drug abusers and (*see*
Intravenous drug abusers)
and economy (162)
employment discrimination and
(145-148)
experimental drugs and
(167-169)
federal assistance programs for
those with AIDS (178)
Finland, prevalence in (151)
France, prevalence in (151)
fungal infections and (30-32)
future growth of cases (161)
Generalized Lymphadenopathy
Syndrome and (44-45)
Haiti, prevalence in (151)
Haitians (*see* Haitians)
health care workers and risk of
acquiring AIDS (*see* Health
care)
hepatitis B vaccine as a means to
acquire AIDS (81)
heterosexuals and (*see*
Heterosexuals)
homosexuals and (*see*
Homosexuals)
household contacts of persons
with AIDS (126)
immunoglobulin injections as a
means to acquire AIDS (82)
infection with virus causing
AIDS (*see* Antibody
positivity)
information centers and AIDS
(179)
intravenous drug abusers and
(*see* Intravenous drug
abusers)

Japan, prevalence in (151)
Kaposi's sarcoma (*see* Kaposi's sarcoma)
lesbians and (57)
money approved for research on (164–166)
monkeys and (*see* Monkeys)
mouth-to-mouth resuscitation as a means of acquiring (131)
nervous system and (34, 35)
Netherlands, prevalence in (151)
Norway, prevalence in (151)
origin of (25)
pneumonia and (32)
prisoners (*see* Prisoners)
prognosis of patients (37–38)
prostitutes (*see* Prostitutes)
protozoan infections and (30–32)
quality of life of persons with AIDS (39)
quarantine and AIDS (144)
recommendations to decrease risk of acquiring AIDS (120, 123, 124, 128)
research institutions (175)
risk of acquiring AIDS for those in no risk group (159)
scientific information sources and AIDS (181)
Singapore, prevalence in (151)
spermicides as protection against AIDS (123)
Sweden, prevalence in (151)
Switzerland, prevalence in (151)
symptoms (26–34)
syndromes of AIDS (27)
Thailand, prevalence in (151)
transmission of AIDS virus
    through artificial insemination (134, 140)
    through blood (84, 139, 140)
    through breast milk (69, 140)
    through casual contact (71–74, 140)
    through contact with urine (140)
    through hepatitis B vaccine (81)
    through immunoglobulin injections (82)
    through insect bites (88, 89)
    through kissing (73, 140)
    through mosquito bites (88, 89)
    through protein injections (83)
    through saliva (72, 73, 131, 132, 140)
    through semen (54, 55, 140)
    through swimming pools or spas (72)
    through tears (129, 140)
    through touching (71–74, 140)
    through transplanted organs (138)
    through vaginal secretions (60–62, 140)
transplant recipients and AIDS (138)
tuberculosis and AIDS (31, 115)
United Kingdom, prevalence in (151)
viral infections and (30–32)
virus causing AIDS (13–14)
West Germany, prevalence in (151)
Acute infection, definition of syndrome (26, 47)
American Federation for AIDS Research (AMFAR) (176)
Antibody negativity
    significance of (101–104)
    infectivity to others of a person who is antibody negative (102–104)
Antibody positivity
    and birth defects in infants (68)
    and breast feeding (69)
    and children (67)
    definition of syndrome (46)
    and ELISA test (97–99)
    family planning in individual having antibody positivity (111)
    immune functioning (115)
    increasing incidence of (121)
    infants and (68)

infectivity to others of person who is antibody positive (106)

interval between antibody positivity and development of AIDS (106–108)

legality of housing and employment discrimination (145–149)

legality of requiring employee to test status (147, 148)

life insurance and (116)

mass screening to determine status (100)

medical evaluation of individuals having (93)

military testing for (118)

organ donation and (119, 138)

precautions to individuals having (111)

prediction of risk of acquiring AIDS (107–110)

pregnancy (111–113, 137)

prevalence among different risk groups (117)

sites to test status (94)

tests used to assess (96–98)

accuracy of tests (95–98)

meaning of tests (99–104)

vaccination of children who are antibody positive (70)

and Western blot test (97–98)

ARC (see Acquired Immunodeficiency-Related Syndrome)

Blood

and transmissibility of AIDS (84)

Blood donation

determination of donor's antibody status (91, 92, 95)

donation facilities as sites for antibody testing (94)

individuals who should avoid blood donation (85)

risk of acquiring AIDS through blood donation (86)

and screening for AIDS virus (91)

Breast milk, transmissibility of AIDS virus (69)

Carrier, asymptomatic carrier of AIDS virus (64, 106)

Casual contact

definition (72)

transmissibility of AIDS virus and casual contact (72–74)

Children with AIDS

breakdown of risk groups (51)

modes of acquiring AIDS (67, 68)

number with AIDS (51)

percentage of AIDS cases (51)

recommendations regarding attendance at school (141, 142)

Drugs, and use against viruses (18, 167–170)

Epidemiology

geography of non-U.S. cases (150–152)

geography of U.S. cases (158)

number of non-U.S. cases of AIDS (151–153)

Ethical dilemmas (184, 185)

FDA, approval for drug research (173, 174)

Generalized Lymphadenopathy Syndrome (GLS)

definition of syndrome (44)

prognosis (45)

relationship to AIDS (45)

Haitians, and AIDS (90)

Health care workers

accidental self-innoculation with contaminated needle (128)

means of acquiring AIDS (125)

protection to decrease risk of acquiring AIDS (127)

right to request AIDS antibody status of a patient (130)

risk of acquiring AIDS (125)

Hemophiliacs

definition (75)

number with AIDS cases (51)

percentage of AIDS cases (51)

prevalence of antibody positivity (78, 79, 117)

prevention of AIDS in (77, 80)

risk of acquiring AIDS (78)

role in AIDS epidemic (76)

use of clotting factor (75, 76)

use of cryoprecipitate (77)

Heterosexuals

changes in sexual behavior (121, 122)

mode of virus spread (54, 55, 56, 60)

number with AIDS (51)

percentage of AIDS cases (51, 62)

percentage related to sexual contact (62)

prevention of AIDS (120, 123)

risk of acquiring AIDS (58)

HIV (*see* Virus, causing AIDS)

Homosexuals

changes in sexual behavior (122)

decreasing the risk of virus transmission to others (111)

initial appearance of AIDS in (52)

mode of virus spread (53–56)

number with AIDS (51)

percentage of AIDS cases (51)

prevalence of antibody positivity (117)

role in spread of AIDS to Europe (63)

HTLV-III (*see* Virus, causing AIDS)

Immune system

definition (3)

effect of AIDS virus on (16, 17)

immune stimulants (17)

Infectivity, of those with AIDS virus exposure (*see* Antibody positivity)

Information and resource centers (179)

Intravenous drug abusers

number with AIDS (51)

percentage of AIDS cases (51)

prevalence of antibody positivity (117)

role in spreading AIDS (65, 66, 67)

shooting galleries (66)

Kaposi's sarcoma

causative agent of (36)

definition (36)

frequency in persons with AIDS (36)

and relationship to diagnosis of AIDS (8, 36)

LAV (*see* Virus, causing AIDS)

Lesbians, and AIDS (57)

Monkeys, and immunodeficiency viruses (22, 25)

Opportunistic infections

and AIDS (30–32)

definition (2)

frequency in persons with AIDS (32)

minimizing the risk of persons with AIDS acquiring infections (33)

organisms causing (30, 31)

sites of opportunistic infections (31)

therapy against (30)

Oral sex, and transmissibility of AIDS (55)

Prisoners, and AIDS (59)

Prostitutes

and AIDS (61)

prevalence of antibody positivity (117)

Rectal sex, and transmissibility of AIDS (56)

Research
 donations for (175–177)
 funding for AIDS research (164–166)
 location of research centers (175)
 private foundations (176)
 resource centers for AIDS information (179)

Saliva, transmissibility of AIDS or virus (73, 131, 132, 140)
Semen, transmissibility of AIDS or virus (54, 134, 140)
Simian Acquired Immuno-deficiency Syndrome (SAIDS) (22, 25)
Syndrome, definition (5)

Tears, transmissibility of AIDS virus (129, 140)

Vaccines
 and viruses (19)
 difficulty of construction (20)
 hepatitis B vaccine and transmission of AIDS (81)
Vaginal secretions, transmissibility of AIDS virus (60, 61, 140)
Virus, AIDS
 acute infection with the AIDS virus (see Acute infection)

affinity of AIDS virus for lymphocytes (13)
affinity of AIDS virus for the nervous system (34, 35)
and antibody (see Antibody positivity)
antiviral drugs (18, 167–170)
asymptomatic carrier of AIDS virus (see Carrier)
definition of (10, 13)
disinfecting techniques (135)
effect of experimental drugs on (167–170)
exposure to AIDS virus (see Antibody positivity)
Human immunodeficiency virus (HIV) (13)
Human T-cell lymphotrophic virus (HTLV-III) (13)
initial appearance in nature (23–25)
Lymphadenopathy-associated virus (LAV) (13)
origin of AIDS virus in humans (25)
sites of virus isolation in body fluids (140)
transmissibility of AIDS virus (see AIDS, transmissibility)
and vaccines (19, 20)
Viruses
 definition (10)
 types of diseases caused by (12)

About the Authors

LYN ROBERT FRUMKIN is a graduate of the University of Washington, where he obtained a combined MD/PhD degree. His postgraduate medical training has been at Stanford University and the University of California at Los Angeles, where he is currently in the Department of Neurology.

JOHN M. LEONARD is a graduate of the University of Wisconsin. He received his MD degree from Johns Hopkins University, and did his postgraduate medical training at Stanford University. Dr. Leonard is currently at the National Institute of Allergy and Infectious Diseases, National Institute of Health, Bethesda, MD, where he is involved in research on AIDS.